Computer Resources
for
People with Disabilities

Support

The production of Computer Resources for People with Disabilities was an exciting experience that demanded a great deal of time and energy on the part of many knowledgeable people throughout the Alliance for Technology Access community. It was a dynamic collaboration of consumers, families, professionals, community-based organizations, technology companies, foundations, and sponsors. We are very grateful to the following companies and foundations for their sponsorship and help in making this effort a success and in promoting the dissemination of this work:

THE MORRIS STULSAFT FOUNDATION

NEC FOUNDATION OF AMERICA

MICROSOFT CORPORATION

MILBANK FOUNDATION FOR REHABILITATION

AUTODESK, INC.

BREGANTE + COMPANY, LLP

ABLENET, INC.

ALPHASMART, INC.

INCLUSIVE TLC

KEYBOWL, INC.

PRENTKE ROMICH COMPANY

TEXTHELP! SYSTEMS LTD.

Praise for
Computer Resources for People with Disabilites

"An Outstanding Academic Book of 1995."
> — Choice *magazine*

"This book on assistive technology speaks directly to people with disabilities and their families. Technology is vital for attaining independence. This book can assist you in finding out how to get it into your life."
> — Ed Roberts, *late president and cofounder, World Institute on Disability*

"This book gets beyond the jargon, beyond the commercialism, and beyond the theory to address the real needs of people with disabilities who want to use technology in their lives."
> — Vicki Casella, Ph.D., *professor, Department of Special Education, San Francisco State University*

"The Alliance for Technology Access has produced an indispensable guide for anyone interested in using computers or assistive technology to expand their horizons in employment, education, or any other area of their lives.... If you're ready to take the plunge into the world of computers, but lack the courage or the knowledge to dive into untested water, *Computer Resources for People with Disabilities* can teach anyone with any kind of disability how to scan, select, and scroll with the best of them."
> — One Step Ahead, a *newsletter by people with disabilities for people with disabilities*

"This wonderful book is another example of the power of parents to change the world. Less than 10 years ago, a few parents recognized that technology could help their children with disabilities. They began a collaborative effort which became the Alliance for Technology Access. Today, these centers serve thousands of children and adults with disabilities, parents, and professionals."
> — Exceptional Parent

"This well-organized work is an invaluable and much-needed reference tool for all types of users.... In this time of universal ADA compliance, this is a highly recommended reference."
> — Library Journal *(starred review)*

"This book is a veritable clearinghouse of the different technologies available and their applicability to the lives and tasks of people with various disabilities. It strives to be a sort of *Whole Earth Catalog* of cutting-edge and approaching technologies.... [It is] informative and unusually easy to use."
— Booklist

"Assistive technology can be liberating, creating opportunities and independence for people with disabilities. This comprehensive and clear guide through the often confusing maze of technology can inform people, and empower them as well."
— *Joseph P. Shapiro, senior editor,* U.S. News & World Report, *and author of* No Pity: People with Disabilities Forging a New Civil Rights Movement

"This book takes the reader step by step through the process of setting goals, assessing needs, finding the right people to help, and getting funding, through the selection of hardware and software to actual purchase and follow-up assistance.... For anyone with a disability or working with a person with a disability, this is probably one of the best starting points to consideration of adapted computer technology. As stated in the book, though, this will only be the start. Where each individual goes will be determined by his/her own needs, desires, and will to succeed and grow."
— Kliatt

"The authors of this book give 'non-techie' people with disabilities (and people who love and work with them) a user-friendly manual for approaching, evaluating, securing, and using computers and assistive devices—all in understandable, simple language."
— Inside MS, *a publication of the National Multiple Sclerosis Society*

"The next time someone says, 'I think a computer would benefit me (my child, my student, my client)—but I don't know where to start,' give them *Computer Resources for People with Disabilities*.... If you can only afford one book, this is probably it."
— Real Times

"There have been many attempts to justify the ways of the 'computer gods' to man. Relatively few of these efforts have addressed assistive technology. What has been missing is a serious and reasonably complete guide for the nonspecialist and the non-professional. Very simply, this is that book."
– *Hod Gray, director, Special Needs Project*

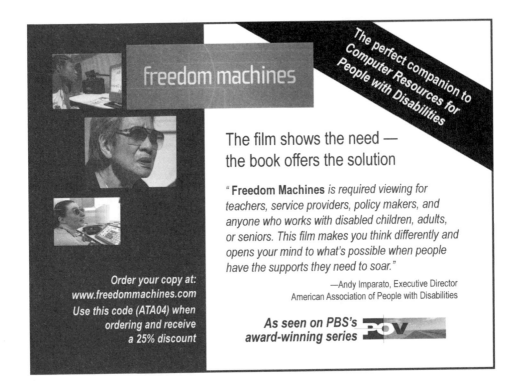
Ordering

Trade bookstores in the U.S. and Canada please contact:

Publishers Group West
1700 Fourth Street, Berkeley CA 94710
Phone: (800) 788-3123   Fax: (510) 528-3444

Hunter House books are available at bulk discounts for textbook course adoptions; to qualifying community, health-care, and government organizations; and for special promotions and fund-raising. For details please contact:

Special Sales Department
Hunter House Inc., PO Box 2914, Alameda CA 94501-0914
Phone: (510) 865-5282   Fax: (510) 865-4295
E-mail: sales@hunterhouse.com

Individuals can order our books from most bookstores, by calling **(800) 266-5592,** or from our website at **www.hunterhouse.com**

Computer Resources for People with Disabilities

A Guide to Assistive Technologies,
Tools and Resources
for People of All Ages

4th Edition

The Alliance for Technology Access

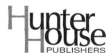

Hunter House
PUBLISHERS

Hunter House Inc., Publishers
PO Box 2914
Alameda CA 94501-0914

Library of Congress Cataloging-in-Publication Data

Computer resources for people with disabilities : a guide to assistive technologies, tools and resources for people of all ages / Alliance for Technology Access.--4th ed.
    p. cm.
    Prev. ed. has title: Computer and web resources for people with disabilities. 3rd ed. © 2000.
    Includes bibliographical references and index.
    ISBN 0-89793-433-4 (pbk.)—ISBN 0-89793-434-2 (spiral bound)
1. Computers and people with disabilities. 2. Computers and people with disabilities—Equipment and supplies. 3. Web site development. I. Computer and web resources for people with disabilities.
HV1569.5.A45 2004
004'.087—dc22   2004002782

Project Credits

Cover Design: Jil Weil, Jinni Fontana
Book Production: Hunter House
Copy Editor: Kelley Blewster
Proofreader: John David Marion
Indexer: Nancy D. Peterson
Acquisitions Editor: Jeanne Brondino
Editor: Alexandra Mummery
Publishing Assistant:
  Alexandra Palmer

Publicist: Lisa E. Lee
Publicity Assistant:
  Gina Kessler
Foreign Rights Assistant:
  Elisabeth Wohofsky
Customer Service Manager:
  Christina Sverdrup
Order Fulfillment: Washul Lakdhon
Administrator: Theresa Nelson
Computer Support: Peter Eichelberger
Publisher: Kiran S. Rana

Printed and Bound by Bang Printing, Brainerd, Minnesota

Manufactured in the United States of America

9 8 7 6 5 4 3   Fourth Edition   06 07 08

Contents

viii

Computer
Resources
for People
with
Disabilities

Dedication

Thomas Oscar Morales (1958–2003) dedicated his life to inclusion, opportunity, dignity, and equity for all people, especially those with disabilities. This book is dedicated to him.

A colleague and friend, Tom approached everything with passion and commitment. He enhanced the power and impact of the Alliance for Technology Access throughout his years with us as a vital member of the team and the community.

Through this book and labor of love, the ATA community honors and thanks Tom for his lasting contribution to our mission, our work, and our lives.

Foreword

This book is about problems of expression and communication and how to solve them. I am dumb, in the literal sense of not being able to speak. Maybe I'm dumb in the more figurative sense, but we won't go into that here. I, and thousands like me, have been helped to communicate by modern technology. Indeed, the fact that I have been asked to write this foreword is a sign of what technology can do.

This book offers something no other does: a guide to maneuvering the growing world of computers, both the mainstream and the assistive technology, to find what is right for you. Evaluating your needs and finding the technology to fill them is a process. My methods of communication are an example.

The main problem of communicating without being able to speak is what is called the *baud rate*, the rate at which information can be conveyed. Normal speech is between 120 and 180 words a minute. By contrast, a reasonable typist can produce 40 to 60 words a minute. Thus, if people were equipped with keyboards to communicate, they could do so at only one-half to one-quarter of the speech rate.

However, many people like me who cannot speak also have other disabilities. They cannot use a keyboard. Instead, they can use one or more switches, operated by a head or hand movement. This is where a person is really confronted with the rate of information flow. If you take an average word to be five characters and assume that any character can follow any other character, normal speech has an information flow rate of between 50 and 75 bits a second. By contrast, a person might be able to operate a switch at two or three bits a second.

The real information flow in human communication, however, is much less than this. (In the case of political speeches, it is practically zero.) This is because spelling out a sentence letter by letter is inefficient. Most sequences of letters don't make recognizable words, let alone meaningful sentences. It takes a handful of these bits of information (letters) to create meaningful communication (a word). So, communicating by specifying every letter is a lot of redundant effort.

For someone who can use a switch to communicate, it is much more efficient to pick words or even whole phrases from a list of likely ones. Computer technology makes this possible. To translate the press of a switch into letters, words, or sentences requires computers. The development of microprocessors in the last 15 years has meant that virtually unlimited computing power is available at a reasonable cost.

The next step is to find efficient software to translate the input from the switch into phrases and sentences. With the Equalizer program that I use, I can manage about 15 words a minute. That is not too bad, since an information flow rate of three bits a second corresponds to 25 to 30 words a minute. But obviously there is scope for improvement. And the promise of computer technology is that improvements are always in development.

Having decoded the signals from some input device, such as a switch, one then has to broadcast it in a form people can understand. This could be visually, with text or diagrams on a screen. But if you want to communicate like others, which is what people in my position would like, you need to be able to speak. Computerized speech synthesizers have improved a great deal in recent years, and this is important: not only does one want to be understood, but one also does not want to sound like Mickey Mouse or a Dalek. My voice may be a bit tinny and American, but it is almost human.

The process I have just described is what this book is all about. I hope others find in this book the inspiration and the technology, hardware and software, that can help them to communicate better—to express their human-ness.

Stephen Hawking
Cambridge University
Cambridge, England

Stephen Hawking is perhaps the best-known modern physicist since Einstein. When he was 21, he was diagnosed with ALS, a degenerative nerve disease. With the use of a voice synthesizer and other computer technology, he has been able to communicate his genius to the world. He is the author of *A Brief History of Time, Black Holes and Baby Universes and Other Essays, The Theory of Everything: The Origin and Fate of the Universe, The Universe in a Nutshell, The Nature of Space and Time, On the Shoulders of Giants,* and others.

Acknowledgments

This book was produced through a collaborative effort of the Alliance for Technology Access, its staff, board, volunteers, friends, and families. The Alliance is a national network dedicated to providing people with disabilities access to technology. The effort that created this book models the Alliance way of doing business. It involves children and adults with disabilities, parents and family members, educators, technology developers, medical professionals, advocates, and friends, all working together to bring the best information and most complete access to interested people everywhere. Most of all, this book is a reflection of the talent within the Alliance, and a tribute to the passion and commitment to our mission.

The Alliance lovingly acknowledges Jackie Brand for her original dream of writing this book. Jackie was the first to inspire us all to contribute our talents and expertise in creating the earliest edition of *Computer Resources for People with Disabilities*. It is under her skillful editing that the fourth edition has taken shape.

The book grew under the loving guidance and tireless efforts of our executive director, Mary Lester. Without her skill, guidance, and patience, this book would not exist. It is Mary's unrivaled commitment to providing assistive-technology resources to families and consumers that has driven the revision of this book.

We are particularly indebted to Bridgett Perry, who coordinated this edition. It was under her fearless leadership that a national team of editors and fact checkers and a dedicated community of assistive-technology experts reshaped the book to meet the needs of today's consumers.

Our utmost appreciation goes to the Alliance staff for their perseverance and commitment during the most difficult of times. The loss of their colleague and friend Tom Morales left every heart broken. Special thanks to Mary Lester, Russ Holland, Libbie Butler, Laura Giacomini, Carol Stanger, and Cindy Flinn for their determination to make this book the best possible in spite of their grief. Their efforts are a tribute to their personal and professional dedication.

We are grateful to Sue Brown for her skill in preparing Part I for the revision. It was her intimate knowledge of the book and her guiding hand that got us off to a great start.

Thank you to Parents Helping Parents, located in Santa Clara, California, and to Through the Looking Glass, located in Berkeley, California, for hosting the focus groups that provided us with critical feedback on the content, design, and approach best able to meet the needs of people with disabilities

xii

Computer
Resources
for People
with
Disabilities

seeking to find the best resources available to them. We are especially grateful to the many participants who shared their impressions and offered invaluable advice.

We acknowledge with great appreciation the wonderful work of graphic designer Sherry Stoll, who helped to create the charts in Part II. We are also grateful to Mary Ann Trower for her hard work and persistence in gathering the photos for this edition.

There are always a few who step up to the plate with every call for help. Among the most generous of heart and mind is Jane Berliss-Vincent. Without her extraordinary contributions, steadfast expertise, and ever-present willingness to do "just one more thing," this edition would never have come to completion. It is also her talent that crafted the Keyword Index, new to this edition. Special appreciation also goes to Lois Symington and Janet Peters for always going the extra mile.

The Alliance would like to acknowledge the hundreds of people who have contributed to the first three editions of this book. Their dedication, hard work, and leadership have provided the core upon which the current edition has been built.

While we cannot possibly name each individual who contributed time and expertise, we wish to thank the many colleagues and friends of the Alliance for their support and knowledge, which is embedded in this work.

Writing Team

Amy Dell, Bridgett Perry, Deborah Newton, Dennis Welton, Helen Miller, Jane Berliss-Vincent, Janet Peters, Janice Fouard, Kathy Reed, Kirsten Haugen, Lisa Wahl, Lois Symington, Marcia J. Scherer, Nancy Stork, Perrine Daily, Robin Stacy

Technical Team

Alice Wershing, Bob Hill, Bridgett Perry, Cindy Mathena, Dennis Welton, Dr. Bob Segalman, Gary King, Holly Roolf, Jane Berliss-Vincent, Janet Nunez, Jenny McGuire, Kathy Griffin, Ken Funk, Linda Bishop Judeich, Linda Rass, Lois Symington, Michelle Laramie, Molly Littleton, Perrine Dailey, Sarah Mak

Fact Checkers

Cathleen Varner, Cindy Mathena, Diane Dew, Harriet Gaston, Jane Berliss-Vincent, Jean Nelson, Jean Wunder, Joanne Castellano, Jonathan Cruce, Julia Petchey, Laura Giacomini, Linda Rass, Mary Ann Trower, Pat Cashdollar, Michelle Laramie

Other Contributors

Alan Bern, Amon Armstrong, Anthony Mercandetti, Anthony Arnold, Carol Stranger, David Clark, Dmitri Belser, Ellen Perlow, Froma Cummings, Helen Miller, Hod Gray, Jane Berliss-Vincent, Jeanette Dodds, Karen Clay, Lynne Cutler, Tom Morales

Reviewers

Alice Wershing, Gary King, Jane Berliss-Vincent, Lisa Wahl

Key Contributors

The following people took key responsibility for the coordination and writing of a chapter in Part I. We thought you might wish to know a bit more about their background and expertise, so we've included a very brief introduction to each of these talented individuals. The breadth and depth of their professional and personal experiences is clearly reflected throughout this edition.

Jane Berliss-Vincent

Jane Berliss-Vincent is director of adult/senior services for the Center for Accessible Technology (CforAT), one of the original Alliance for Technology Access centers, in Berkeley, California. Her prior jobs in the assistive-technology field included working for vendors and research organizations.

Jackie Brand

Jacquelyn Brand was the founder and first executive director of the Alliance for Technology Access. Her work grew out of a personal challenge to find appropriate technology for her daughter, Shoshana. She is the founder and president of Independent Living Network, a nonprofit organization dedicated to developing options for independent living for individuals with disabilities.

Perrine Daily

Perrine Dailey has been an assistive-technology specialist at PACER's Simon Technology Center since 1995. Perrine has a profound hearing loss and wears hearing aids. She presents workshops and in-services, conducts consultations for children and adults with disabilities, manages the software and device loan library, and writes for national publications.

xiv

Computer
Resources
for People
with
Disabilities

Amy Dell

Amy Dell is a professor of special education at the College of New Jersey, where she serves as director of the Adaptive Technology Center for New Jersey Colleges, an ATA affiliate, and the Center on Assistive Technology and Inclusive Education Studies, an ATA resource center.

Janice Fouard

Janice Fouard has worked with assistive technology since 1989. She provides direct services and information and referral. She recently began working with the Kansas AgriAbility Program at OCCK, Inc.

Kirsten Haugen

Kirsten Haugen, based in Eugene, Oregon, is a freelance consultant for educational and assistive technology. She is a major contributor to the ATA's Family Place in Cyberspace website and coauthor of "We Can Play," a series of free accessible-play ideas in English and Spanish, also available at the ATA website.

Helen Miller

Helen Miller has been a special-education teacher for 28 years, a college lecturer, and a presenter at many special-education conferences. She has worked for 15 years in the field of assistive technology, and for 13 years, collaboratively, at the Center for Accessible Technology as a consultant specialist in assistive technology in education.

Deborah Newton

Deborah Newton is currently an assistant professor in the Department of Special Education, Language, and Literacy at the College of New Jersey, where she teaches courses in assistive technology (AT) and other subjects. She has extensive experience as an assistive-technology specialist and continues to provide AT training workshops and AT assessments.

Bridgett Perry

Bridgett Perry specializes in community technology, education technology, and assistive technology for people with disabilities. She is the owner of Perry and Associates, a consulting business that helps community-based organizations plan and implement programs and services. Bridgett is the creator and leader of the CITTI Project (Community Inclusion Through Technology, International), which provides assistive-technology support for communities in developing countries.

Janet Peters

Janet Peters has been the director of PACER's Simon Technology Center since 1994. Her background includes a decade of direct service with families. She has developed and presented courses in national technology, is the managing editor for *Computer Monitor*, and has coordinated several federally funded grant projects. She has a background in computer science and organizational communication.

Kathy Reed

Kathy Reed has worked in the assistive-technology field since 1994. She currently directs the Technology Resource Solutions for People assistive technology program at OCCK, Inc., one of the original Alliance for Technology Access sites (ATA).

Marcia J. Scherer, Ph.D.

Marcia Scherer directs the Institute for Matching Person and Technology and is senior research associate at the International Center for Hearing and Speech Research (National Technical Institute for the Deaf/Rochester Institute of Technology) and associate professor of physical medicine and rehabilitation, University of Rochester Medical Center. She has written books and articles on assistive technology from a user's perspective.

Robin Stacy

Robin Stacy earned a bachelor of arts degree in special education from the University of Kentucky and a master of education degree from the University of Louisville. After teaching for five years, she now works for Enabling Technologies of Kentuckiana, where she helps persons with disabilities implement assistive technology into their daily lives.

Nancy Stork

Nancy Stork has provided direct services and information and referral services with the assistive-technology program at OCCK, Inc., since 1992. She received her certification as an assistive-technology practitioner in 2002. Before that, she worked at OCCK as a certified sign-language interpreter.

Lois Symington

Lois Symington is a teacher, college professor, ATA center director, and parent of a 29-year-old son with disabilities. Her desire to find better ways of teaching all children provided the impetus for exploring uses of technology in teaching and learning.

xvi

Computer
Resources
for People
with
Disabilities

Lisa Wahl

Lisa Wahl has spent the past 23 years working with agencies that serve people with disabilities, including 10 years at the Center for Accessible Technology. While she finds most legislation tedious, she has become extremely enthused about the possibilities of Section 508 for education (the Rehabilitation Act that requires federal agencies to make their electronic and information technology accessible to people with disabilities).

Dennis Welton

Dennis Welton holds a bachelor of science degree in biomedical engineering and a master of science degree in systems engineering/rehabilitation engineering from Wright State University, in Dayton, Ohio. His professional career in assistive technology has spanned a period of 10 years and four states. He has worked for state governments, in private business, and for nonprofit centers. Currently he is at the STAR Center, a nonprofit rehabilitation center and a member of the Alliance for Technology Access.

The Alliance is deeply grateful to Hunter House. Without their belief and trust in us, we would not have had this tremendous opportunity to share with you what we have learned. We especially appreciate their commitment to promoting access for consumers, family members, and professionals everywhere.

Our work, though utterly fascinating and truly compelling, has rarely been confined to a mortal's time schedule, as all of our wonderful and significant others will unanimously agree. Among the most important contributors have been and continue to be our own families, who often and gracefully handle the personal loads that allow us to follow our dreams.

Most importantly, we thank the people we meet every day in every center who have taught us so much and who have, in countless ways, contributed to the richness of this book.

Important Note to the Reader

The material in this book is intended to provide an overview of the hardware, software, and other considerations surrounding computer resources for people with disabilities. Every effort has been made to provide accurate and dependable information, and the contents of this book have been compiled in consultation with a variety of computer professionals and users. The reader should be aware that professionals in the field may have differing opinions and that change is always taking place. Therefore, the authors, publisher, and editors cannot be held responsible for any error, omission, or outdated material.

The authors and publisher disclaim any liability, loss, injury, or damage incurred as a consequence, directly or indirectly, of the use and application of any of the contents of this volume.

Many of the designations used by manufacturers and sellers to distinguish their products are claimed as trademarks. Where those designations appear in this book, and the authors were aware of a trademark claim, the designations have been printed with initial capital letters. The inclusion of a product in this book does not imply endorsement or recommendation.

The people and events described in the personal stories in this book are real. In some cases, their names have been changed to respect their privacy and that of their families.

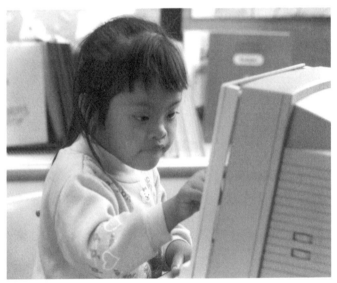

Introduction

Since the first edition of this book was released in 1994, everyone's expectations for technology have increased exponentially. The resources and tools available to both people with and people without disabilities have multiplied dramatically. Imagining how technology can enhance life is something more and more of us do regularly. As the tools become increasingly sophisticated, it is easier to think about customizing a computer to make it work specifically for us. We know we can get a computer to talk to us. We know that keyboards come in a wide range of types and sizes. We know we can walk up to a computer, such as an ATM, touch its screen, and have it respond. We know we can access the information on hundreds of millions of computers around the globe from home by connecting to the Internet.

As the general public's expectations for technology have risen, so have those of people with disabilities. For someone with a disability or functional limitation, today's applications offer incredible promise and excitement. The technology currently on the market can provide access to employment, education, and leisure activities. It can support increased independence at home and in the community. It provides a means for communication and civic participation.

Keyboards are available that change effortlessly from a standard layout to one that includes only the keys you need for a specific task, such as creating a budget, working on an English assignment, or exploring music composition. Talking computers can read you mail sent from around the world, enable you to shop online, and help you withdraw cash from your local ATM. You can file your tax return electronically without using your hands, simply by looking at the right letters on a keyboard pictured on the computer screen.

These are just of few examples of what you can do with technology today. The promise of technology for people with disabilities is unlimited. Realizing that promise takes a lot of information, advice, and support, all of which we have endeavored to provide in this book.

Why This Book Was Written

If you are a person with a disability, or if you are a parent, other family member, teacher, employer, or friend of a person with a disability, we want to share with you what we have learned about the ways assistive technology changes lives by creating new abilities for children and adults with disabilities and functional limitations—whether those limitations be sensory, cognitive, learning, or physical.

Every day, in the course of our work, we are asked questions about available technology and its applications: "I have a vision impairment. Which computer should I buy?" "My son has a learning disability, and his teacher said a computer might help him do better in school. Which should I buy?" "I have a girl in my sixth-grade class with cerebral palsy, and the school has agreed to provide her with a computer. Which is the best?" Your questions may be similar.

The goal of *Computer Resources for People with Disabilities* is to help you answer your questions and to allow you to take advantage of the incredible tools on the market today. We won't teach you about the workings of the latest computers or list every computer product ever developed. Our intention is to help you create a plan and a framework for approaching technology so you can make initial decisions about the role it can play in your life. We have included many stories about real people who are using technology successfully—people of all ages and all kinds of disabilities who use technology for different reasons.

This book was written for a community that has much to gain from the power of technology. The community includes people with disabilities, but it also includes family members, advocates, and friends of people with disabilities. It includes thousands of professionals in the fields of education and rehabilitation who are concerned about quality-of-life issues and options for children and adults with disabilities. It includes technologists, engineers, and designers who will be the developers of tomorrow's technology. This broad group represents a huge constituency that is being dramatically impacted by technology in this century. We believe this constituency will undergo nothing less than a revolution in expectations, making even more options available for people with disabilities everywhere.

Throughout the book, we address the audience as "you," in recognition of the important decision-making role played by individuals with disabilities in defining their own futures. Supportive family members, friends, advocates, and professionals should translate the wording as needed, but always remember that choices about technology should be, to the greatest possible degree, dictated by the user.

A Word about Us

We, the authors, are a diverse group of people who have become connected and interrelated by our search for technologies to support our dreams. We are people with disabilities, children and adults, family members and friends, teachers and therapists, employers, service providers, advocates, technology vendors, professional organizations, and community agencies. We come from all over the United States, from small towns and urban centers. We cross age, ethnic, and ability/disability lines. We represent a growing community of people across the country and around the globe who are employing the tools of technology and reaching new levels of satisfaction. We did not choose technology because we were intrinsically interested in it; we became users of technology because it allowed us to become what we wanted to be: teachers, communicators, artists, composers, students, and engineers.

We are connected by a strong belief in the vast potential of people with disabilities to use technology to achieve their dreams, and by a profound commitment to bringing the benefits of technology to people who have historically been excluded from the American dream. We have been through the process of trying to understand a bewildering and complex field. We have searched for expertise and support. And we have created an organization, the Alliance for Technology Access, that bonds us to each other and to all people looking for similar answers and support.

The Alliance for Technology Access is a collaborative, energetic community of people redefining what it means to have a disability. Having a disability no longer has to mean that things cannot be done; it means that we can find new ways to get them done. The Alliance is made up of expert advocates dedicated to pushing the limits of convention—people who ask not whether something can be done, but rather how it can be accomplished. We share your challenges and your frustrations. We believe in every person's right to be productive and independent and to achieve his or her desired quality of life. And we believe the most noble application of technology is to support that right.

The Alliance is a network of assistive-technology resource centers, consumer groups, technology programs, individuals, and technology vendors. Our members share a common vision: an uncommon commitment to improving the quality of life for children and adults with disabilities and functional limitations through the imaginative application of technology.

The Alliance was created to demonstrate how technology can transform limitations into opportunities. We work toward this goal by providing access to assistive technologies and related services that enable people to achieve productivity, independence, and success according to their individual needs and interests.

People with disabilities must be at the heart of the learning and decision-making process. We take an approach to service, both at our centers and in this book, that varies from the standard, professionally driven model that assumes the "experts" know what's best for you. We believe that we as individuals know what we need; that a team that includes professional resources can help guide us in the right direction; and that, in the end, we must make our own decisions and direct our own lives.

The Structure of the Book

Computer Resources for People with Disabilities, like the Alliance, represents a collaborative effort, with many voices adding richness and texture to the content. We represent a great diversity of approaches and solutions, each with its own purpose and validity. We will introduce you to a broad and growing community of technology users who are excited and eager to share what they have learned.

You may find the arrangement of this book somewhat unusual. Many books relating to people with disabilities are arranged according to disability. You can usually turn to a chapter on "visual impairments" or "physical disabilities," and you are likely to read about a particular tool that was designed for a specific disability.

We focus instead on tools for getting better access to the environment, regardless of your particular disability. We know that a well-designed environment or an excellent set of tools to navigate around barriers can make all the difference.

We also look at technology through the lens of an individual's strengths and functional abilities and limitations, rather than through his or her disability. In this way, we are able to suggest tools and strategies that build on strengths and maximize function. If the goal is to have a screen display large letters, it doesn't really matter if you need it because you have a visual impairment, a learning disability, or some other impairment. The question is not what does a person with X disability require, but rather what are the ways in which we can enlarge print on a computer screen.

Based on feedback from readers of earlier editions, we have added a Keyword Index to this edition to help you find what you need more readily. The Keyword Index will help you find information relevant to your particular functional limitation and relevant to your specific goals and most immediate questions. Although the book as a whole is not structured around categories of disability or functional limitation, we recognize the need to reference such categories as a useful way to retrieve information. Through the Keyword Index, this edition provides the opportunity to quickly and easily check out all references to your particular disability.

The book is divided into three parts. Part I, "The Search for Solutions," will guide you through the process of defining your needs, developing a technology plan, building a supportive team, and making technology-related decisions. It offers strategies, first steps, and resources, and it should help you become more confident in your exploration.

Part I has been completely revised in this edition to offer you the latest information in a direct and easy-to-read format. Each of the nine chapters covers a phase of the technology-planning process, and each chapter has been written by a different expert or team of experts.

Another change in this edition is that each chapter in Part I includes a section devoted to providing you with information based on your particular life situation. Your life situation provides the context for using technology, whether it involves employment, school, or community, or relates to issues of aging, injury, or illness. All of these life experiences will naturally affect your technology-planning process and decisions, and, as such, all are discussed in the book.

Each of the chapters in Part I also includes new worksheets and checklists. These are meant to guide you through your planning process. They may be photocopied and used to track your decisions and directions. They will help you keep your goals in mind as you go through the various planning phases. If you like, you can go straight to the chapters that are relevant to your current needs without reading through all the chapters in the order in which they are presented. You can enter the planning process from any point, depending on your knowledge, comfort level, and goals.

Part II, "The Technology Toolbox," focuses on the technology itself by listing examples of various assistive technologies. It will inform and direct your search by helping you to zero in on the technologies most likely to match your abilities and goals. Part II can be read selectively as you narrow your search. It is not a compendium of every product on the market, but through it you will learn enough about the categories of products available today to feel comfortable taking the next steps.

The search for technology solutions is a lifelong process. As your life changes and as technology evolves, you'll find yourself looking for new and better solutions. That is one of the most exciting aspects of this field: realizing that technology is constantly evolving. Changes are so rapid that information is often out-of-date before it is printed. We can't predict your needs or the products that will be available in the future, but we can provide you with a plan and with appropriate resources for starting and continuing your search. You may find yourself referring to "The Technology Toolbox" again and again whenever you consider new options.

Part III, "Helpful Resources and References," contains lists of resources, references, and organizations that we have found valuable in our personal and professional study of assistive technology. Keep in mind that as quickly as the technology changes, so does the information regarding the players in this newly emergent field.

This fourth edition includes a great deal of updated information, and since the Internet is such a powerful vehicle for the delivery of ever-changing information, we plan to utilize it to maintain updates about what we are sharing in this book. We encourage you to continue your search via our website at www.ATAccess.org.

Much of what we offer in this book are the right questions for you to ask and some key resources to help you find the answers to those questions. You will learn how others have faced challenges similar to yours and have developed effective strategies. You will hear a lot about planning and process, pursuit and persistence, goals and rights, exploration and community. We will go over what you should know, where to go, and what to do next. It is our objective to present you with sound advice and guidance to assist you in finding the tools you need to realize your dreams. We have accomplished that objective if, after reading this book, you have a goal in mind, an idea about some easy first steps to take toward reaching that goal, and a range of supporters to help you. We have also accomplished our objective if you come away from reading this book armed with enough information to talk comfortably with your local computer dealer, or if you are inspired or excited by someone's story. We wish you great success in your ventures into the world of assistive technology.

Part I

The Search for Solutions

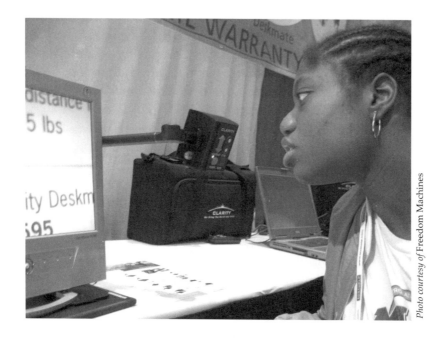

Chapter 1

Creating a Vision

Why Do I Need a Plan?

*Lois Symington, Ph.D., executive director of the East Tennessee
Technology Access Center, Knoxville, Tennessee*

The Big Picture

Some say that the one constant in the twenty-first century is change. That is
certainly true when we contemplate the role of technology and the impact of
disability in our lives. In the face of constant and inevitable change, we
quickly realize that one way of coping is to create a vision of what we want to
accomplish. A personal vision can serve as a sort of map or guide. This chapter will help you begin developing a vision for acquiring and using the technology that is suitable for you.

Begin by thinking about your personal goals and the ways that technology can help you reach those goals. As you do, keep in mind the constant
change with which you'll be faced. As we reach different phases or ages in
our lives, our needs change as a natural part of growing up and growing
older. Some types of disabilities cause fluctuating changes in mobility, hearing, vision, and cognition. Technology also changes daily, and we are constantly bombarded with information about the newest and latest gadget that
is more intuitive, smaller, and faster than the last. The technology described
in this book provides unprecedented opportunities—at home, at school, in
the workplace, and in the community—for people with disabilities. With
today's exciting new tools, existing stereotypes and assumptions about having a disability can be tossed out in favor of new expectations and greater
integration into all facets of life.

Because of ongoing and dramatic shifts in technology, we do not need to
be limited in our thinking about what is available today. For this reason, we
encourage you to start with a vision of what *can be* rather than what *is*. If
someone can dream it, someone else will design, adapt, modify, develop, or
make it. We should also avoid limiting our thinking to high-tech Dick
Tracy–type technology. A place mat comprised of communication symbols or
a one-message communication device might be as effective in delivering the
message "please pass the salt" as a more expensive or sophisticated device.

The role of technology is to support and enhance human relationships, to provide access to new things or to old things in new ways, to unleash human potential, and to redefine power and control. Set your goals high to meet the possibilities of tomorrow's technology.

Using technology to do things for ourselves, rather than depending on people to do things for us, allows us to control our own lives. *Chris,* a young man with cerebral palsy who uses an array of assistive-technology devices to control a computer, says through his communication-software program, "Today I think about my life differently because now I can read and write." Chris had a dream and a plan: to learn to read and write, get a job, and live in his own apartment. As of today, he is halfway there. If he and his family had merely accepted what his teachers and therapists expected of him, he would still be illiterate and have no future apart from one imposed by others.

The focus of this book is to look at the processes and steps we can take to reach our personal goals by incorporating technology into our everyday lives. Some of those aspirations might include reading the newspaper, talking on the telephone, retrieving objects off high shelves, playing with toys, or participating in a math lesson. Because of technology, people who are blind, who cannot stand to reach, who may be unable to use their hands or arms, or who may have difficulty learning in traditional ways can do all these daily activities and more.

Useful Preparation

The words we use can sometimes create barriers to learning about ourselves and our potential. For example, the word *technology* usually creates an image of a computer, robot, or Palm Pilot. When we add words like *assistive* or *adaptive,* people may become increasingly confused and wonder if the phrase really has anything to do with them. Some cultures may even lack words for *assistive technology* or familiarity with the concept. Likewise, the notion that technology can provide freedom and autonomy may be viewed differently from one culture or community to another. To make sure that we, the authors of this book, are "speaking the same language" as you, the reader, we have defined a few words and phrases commonly used when discussing technology solutions.

Conventional technology

We consider the term *conventional technology* to mean typical computers and their operating systems and programs. These are the products that are readily found in your local computer stores. They are the tools you see everywhere—in offices, schools, libraries, etc. As technology has evolved, so has the capacity of conventional computers and software to flexibly meet the needs of a wide range of users with and without disabilities. Sometimes the technology solution is already built into the computer sitting on your desk. Once you know about these features, they are easily available to you at no extra cost.

Universal design

As conventional technology moves toward being useable by a wider and more diverse group of people, it is described as being *universally designed*. This means that the designer of the piece of equipment or program has taken into account the varying learning styles and needs of potential users. Rather than only being a tool used by someone with a disability, it is a tool that works better for everyone, including someone with a disability. An example is the location of a computer power switch on the keyboard or on the front of the computer. This change from the traditional rear-mounted switch was critical to independent computer use by many people with disabilities and is a great convenience to every computer user.

Assistive-technology device

As defined in the Assistive Technology Act of 1998, the term *assistive-technology device* means any item, piece of equipment, or product system—whether acquired commercially off the shelf, modified, or customized—that is used to increase, maintain, or improve the functional capabilities of people with disabilities. The term *assistive-technology device* is often abbreviated to the words *assistive technology* or the acronym *AT*. You will find these phrases used throughout the book.

An assistive-technology device can be as simple as an adapted spoon, as familiar as a wheelchair, or as complex as an eye-gaze system that controls a computer. The definition of *assistive technology* as originally stated in the Technology-Related Assistance for Individuals with Disabilities Act of 1994 (also known as the Tech Act) has been used in all subsequent legislation, including the Americans with Disabilities Act (ADA), the Amendments to the Rehabilitation Act, and changes to the Individuals with Disabilities Education Act (IDEA). While the reader may incorporate all types of assistive technology into his or her life, this book specifically focuses on computer-related technology solutions.

Assistive-technology services

According to the Tech Act of 1994, an assistive-technology service directly assists a person with a disability in the selection, acquisition, or use of an assistive-technology device.

This same law, for the first time, also recognized the role of the user—that is, the person with a disability—in selecting, acquiring, and using assistive-technology devices. Terms such as *consumer-responsive* helped establish a person-centered model of services that was intended to shift control of devices, services, and funding sources from professionals to users or "consumers" of these devices and services. Other components of assistive-technology services include the right to an evaluation and the right to purchase, lease, or replace devices.

Disability

In U.S. statute 42 U.S.C. § 12102(2), the term *disability* means, with respect to an individual,

(a) a physical or mental impairment that substantially limits one or more of the major life activities of such individual;

(b) a record of such an impairment; or

(c) being regarded as having such an impairment.

Disability is a universally common occurrence and characteristic of the human condition. The U.S. Census Bureau states that in the United States there are 54 million people with disabilities. That represents 20 percent of the population. People with disabilities are the nation's largest minority. As people age, the prevalence of visual, hearing, and mobility disabilities greatly increases. Most people, if they live long enough, will age into disability.

The presence of a disability, whether congenital or acquired through accident, injury, or illness, may have an impact on the type of technology you need and how you develop your plan for acquiring that technology. For example, if you have ALS (amyotrophic lateral sclerosis, or Lou Gehrig's disease), you may need to think in terms of how the technology you use today can be adapted or modified as your needs and abilities change. On the other hand, if you break your arm and can't use your dominant hand to write for three months, you may need some temporary modification in order to continue to use a computer.

Throughout this book we tend to think about disability in terms of function or functional limitation. We are less concerned about any particular disability by name or category than we are about the specific functions you are trying to build or enhance. Access to technology is often the means by which you can accomplish your personal goals. Whether your need for an alternate method of using the computer is due to one disability or another does not matter. We look at how to improve upon your functions or address a functional limitation through a good match with the appropriate device.

Remember Chris, who was mentioned earlier in the chapter? Chris was 18 years old when he first started visiting his local technology-access center in Knoxville, Tennessee. That was eight years ago. He has cerebral palsy, cannot use his voice to speak words, has limited use of his arms and hands, and has difficulty controlling the movements of his body. Chris, along with the staff of the center and Chris's parents, worked as a team toward his dream of getting on the Internet by himself. He was aware of the power of words, but he could not read or write. In his own words (typed recently on a computer with the use of a word prediction program and switch interface), "I didn't want to read and write, but I had to learn to get on the Internet."

Chris continues to work with his team to identify the technology solutions that will enable him to gain the self-confidence, the increased levels of literacy, and the employment skills necessary to create webpages. He

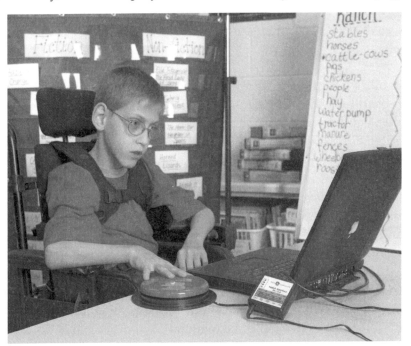

The Don Johnston Switch Interface Pro 5.0 connects up to 5 standard switches to run switch-enabled software from a wide variety of publishers. (Photo courtesy of Don Johnston)

now uses the Internet independently, sends e-mails to friends, and participates in chat rooms. This is a journey that is ongoing, as he and his family cope with his transition from school, obtain support from the state's Medicaid program, attain services through vocational rehabilitation, acquire transportation (no easy task in rural eastern Tennessee), and continue to support his fledgling independence. His technology has changed from an Apple IIE computer (in 1995) to his current setup, a portable system equipped with EZ Keys and augmentative communication software. The changes in his technology were a result of gains in literacy skills, advances in technology, and changes in his personal life.

Steps to Consider

Creating a vision for how you will use technology and then developing a plan to achieve that vision will make the process of gaining access to technology more manageable. Your plan will evolve as you gain more knowledge and deal with issues, such as funding sources, transportation, building a support network, and culturally based differences in expectations. There will be overlapping circles of goals, needs, abilities, technology, and supports and services that shape and modify your plan.

Make a Plan

You do not need to know about existing technology in order to develop plans to achieve your vision. What is more important is for you to determine the things that you want to be able to do that are now difficult or impossible. Is it important for you to read books by yourself, write your own letters, converse on the telephone, play card games with your friends, visit the library each week, or see the recipes you are trying to cook? Would you like to be able to get out of a chair by yourself rather than have to wait for someone to help you? Are books too heavy or impossible for you to carry, hold, or use? Do you want people to understand what you want to say? Chapter 2 will guide you through the planning process.

Know Your Resources

Once you have a vision in mind, examine your financial resources and your "people" resources. Very few of us are born wealthy enough to purchase whatever we want, whenever we want it, which makes us dependent on other funding sources. Some of these funding sources may be mandated by federal law, such as those protecting the rights of infants and children to an equal education, providing support for adults who want to go to work, or setting requirements for accessibility in the workplace. Beyond your own personal resources, private insurance as well as state Medicaid and federal Medicare programs may cover assistive-technology devices that are considered medically necessary. Civic groups, such as Sertoma, the Lions Club, and Kiwanis, as well as churches or charitable individuals or businesses, may provide at least partial funding for needed devices. Chapter 6 is full of ideas and strategies for funding.

People resources may include family members who will help you learn to use or care for a device, as well as therapists and teachers who may want to incorporate the use of a device into a therapy setting or classroom. Vocational rehabilitation counselors may support your need to use assistive technology in job-training classes. Peers and colleagues are also important resources. They may help with transportation so you can get training on the use of your new devices or provide critical moral and technical support during the learning period. Vendors of products are also important people resources, as they may be available to demonstrate or loan new products.

You should also learn about resources in your community. You may have a neighborhood school, community technology center, or Alliance for Technology Access center where you can learn about products or get training. Vendors may offer free or low-cost training in your area. Your local office on aging may have information or resources about low-tech devices that would help you live in your own home more easily or independently. Refer to Chapter 3 for information on developing your people resources.

Know Your Rights and Be Your Own Advocate

Every state in the United States has an independent-living center, a parent-training program, an advocacy service, and free or low-cost legal services. These are available for you to utilize when you feel that you are not getting the devices or services you need. Existing federal laws protect the rights of people with disabilities in the workplace and ensure access to public buildings and programs. Some existing laws are considered civil rights laws, such as the Americans with Disabilities Act. Other laws are considered entitlement legislation because the presence of a disability entitles students, for example, to the same educational experiences as peers without disabilities. Medicare may fund a speech-generating device (SGD) if it is considered a medical necessity; however, actually acquiring a device through Medicare may be contingent on knowing your resources and rights. Chapter 5 will help you learn more about your legal rights.

Know Your Needs and Abilities

Finally, determine your personal needs and abilities in the context of continuous change. A purchase, rental, or loan today may meet a need for a week or a month, and then you may need to look for something else. Today's technology may not even be available six months from now. Using technology to meet personal goals requires continuous assessment of where you are on the path to your goal. Are your needs being met, is the technology meeting your needs, and do you need technical support in terms of more training, repairs, or updates to the product you are using? Just as you would not buy a pair of shoes to last a lifetime, you would not purchase a piece of technology to last a lifetime. Your feet will grow and your preferences will change. Today's technology may not meet tomorrow's needs.

This is *Leah's* story, as told by her mother, Susan. Leah is a 14-year-old who was born prematurely with developmental delays. When she was two years old and not yet speaking, a speech pathologist suggested that the family consider assistive technology and augmentative communication. She also suggested that the family learn about new technologies by attending an assistive-technology exposition. At this event, the family connected with a local technology-access center and had the chance to "look into Leah's future" as she used a computer equipped with a touch screen and various children's programs.

When Leah turned three years old and became eligible for services from the local school system, the family had an assistive-technology plan in place. By this time, Leah's parents had learned two things: The first was to build a foundation of knowledge and skills in order to successfully advocate for needed services. The second was to use that knowledge to develop a plan for Leah that could be presented to the school system. This strategy placed Leah and her family in a proactive rather than reactive position, and led to more productive outcomes for Leah.

Susan offers the following suggestions to those of you who are starting to make plans for obtaining assistive-technology devices and services:

- Get involved with a local technology-access center, such as ATA, if there is one in your community. This will become the foundation from which you access technology, through evaluations, training, one-on-one contact with qualified staff, and the use of the lending library of software and hardware.

- Talk to professionals who are independent. This will enable you to become educated and trained before you sit down with professionals who have power over funding decisions.

- Trust your instincts. You know yourself or your child best. In Susan's words, "We realize that most of our mistakes have occurred when we have not followed our instincts."

- Be prepared for changing needs over time. Technology is constantly changing and is rarely a one-time need.

- Look for training opportunities that keep you abreast of new and exciting technologies. Take advantage of training offered in your community, whether at school, at a local technology-access center, by vendors, at conferences, or online.

- If possible, own the technology you use. You will become more involved in the programming (in the case of, say, a communication device) or setup of your device and have more control over content if you own it rather than lease or borrow it. In Leah's case, it also resulted in pride in ownership.

- Be creative. Learn to piggyback services. There is a shortage of all types of disability services, and there is no one-stop shopping. For Leah, school is only one aspect of her life. She also has a life at home and in the community. Adopt a broader plan, and consider all your local resources.

- Embrace advocacy as part of the process. Leah's parents realized that advocacy is a natural part of interacting with the school system and that formal complaints, mediation, and due process are the advocacy tools provided to parents by law. They began to think of advocacy for assistive technology as a part of their job in acquiring the devices and services that Leah needs.

When Leah and her parents moved to eastern Tennessee, they found the local technology-access center there and continued their "offensive planning" for Leah's future. Susan says, "Through early intervention, the elementary school years, and now into the transition years, our technology-access center has provided us with the direction to maintain a family assistive-technology plan. As we look toward Leah's future as a high school student and then as an adult, we are excited about the prospects that assistive technology will offer her."

How Life Situations Impact Planning for Assistive Technology

Your life situation—that is, your current environment or life circumstances—can greatly impact your assistive-technology plan. Whether you need technology to assist you in school, at work, or at home will influence where you go for funding, what your rights are, and what resources are available to you. Consider the following issues when developing a vision for your technology needs.

Early Childhood

During the early childhood years (birth to three years old) the focus is on children's development in areas such as play, language, cognition, and motor abilities. The purpose of assistive technology for young children with disabilities is to support their needs in these key developmental areas and to provide them with a way to participate with their peers in all activities. Types of technology for young children include adapted toys, simple communication devices, and multisensory toys that allow exploration and self-paced learning. Even at a young age, children with disabilities can learn to control things in their environment and to use simple communication devices to say single words ("Momma"), make requests ("Want ball"), or participate in group activities ("My turn"). The goals for young children are usually written into an individualized family support plan (IFSP), which may also include training for parents and service providers on how to incorporate assistive-technology devices into daily routines at home, at therapy, or in a day-care center. Devices purchased by outside funding, such as that provided under Part C of the Individuals with Disabilities Education Act (IDEA), are the child's property and are generally used at home.

School Years

When children with disabilities turn three years old and until their 22nd birthday, they qualify for a full range of services, as mandated by the IDEA. Some families choose to use private insurance to fund things such as augmentative communication devices or wheelchairs. The law clearly specifies that children with disabilities are to receive the supports and services necessary to obtain an education equal to that of their peers without disabilities. A team that includes parents, teachers, and other support staff develops yearly goals for the child. At each step in the development of the plan, raise the question with the team of whether assistive technology might be a necessary support. The plan should be reviewed on a regular basis to see if the child's needs have changed. An important question to ask is what does the child need in order to participate in the same or equal activities as the child's peers who don't have disabilities?

Transition to Adult Living

If you are a student with disabilities who is exiting high school or approaching the age of 22, your transition to adult services may include support from vocational rehabilitation. A transition plan may have started for you around age 14; in any event, it must be in place by the time you are 16. It's important to allow sufficient time for developing an adequate transition plan. The goals and plans that you develop at this stage in your life should be directed toward answering the following questions: How do I want to live as an adult? Do I want to live alone? Have a job? Drive a car? Receive a college education? Get married? The answers to these questions should form the goals of the transition plan. Other questions to consider include the following: Are you using any assistive-technology devices that are the property of the school? What will happen if you don't have access to them after exiting the school system? Do you need to look at alternate funding sources for these devices?

In 1981, when *Dusty* was just six years old, she visited her friend John and was amazed at all he was doing with his Apple II+ (an early Apple computer). Dusty saw immediately what power John had. Control was an issue for Dusty, as she had Down syndrome and very little control over

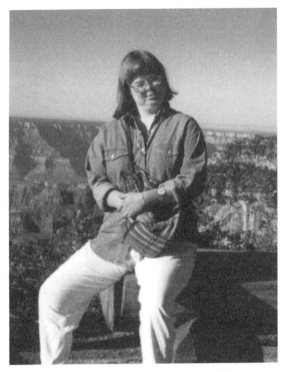

Dusty

things in her life at that time. With John's computer, she could push a button and make things happen. Her parents had to drag her home from that first technology encounter.

Dusty was in a regular kindergarten at the time. Her parents were told that she did not pay attention well and wouldn't stay on task. Her mother knew the trick would be to find a task that would engage Dusty.

Through her research, Dusty's mother learned that children with Down syndrome tend to be good visual learners. That clinched it for her.

At Christmas Dusty's parents bought her an Apple II+ and some intriguing early-learning software programs that explored the alphabet and numbers. Dusty learned the keyboard quickly and began practicing counting without even being encouraged to do so.

Dusty's mother had had no prior experience with computers and wasn't mechanically inclined. She and Dusty learned together. As a way to get her daughter access to a computer at school, she volunteered to help the teacher and work with the other students. As the children used the software, it became clear to the teacher that Dusty could be included in activities using the computer, just like everyone else.

Later, Dusty attended her local high school and took many classes with her nondisabled peers, including a computer class. A word processing program with large print, speech output, and word prediction gave her the support she needed for writing. Using these tools, she wrote children's books in her English class, which she then read to the babies in the day-care center where she worked one period a day.

By age 24, Dusty had completed four years at her local community college. She enjoyed classes in keyboarding, using a computer for personal and business purposes, and using the Internet. Screen magnification software was provided by the college's Disabled Students Program. Soon after college she started her first paying part-time job and continued doing volunteer work. She and her mom built a web page with picture icons representing links to her favorite Internet sites. In that way her web page served as a support system for her.

Independent living (with support) was one of Dusty's goals. When she was focused on learning to cook, she and her mom or helper added new recipes each week to the electronic cookbook she was compiling. Luckily, her standard database software, FileMaker Pro (FileMaker Inc.), included a large-print option, so the support she needed was built in.

As her mother says, "Technology gave Dusty confidence in her ability as a learner. She began to feel good about herself. Her self-esteem improved. Technology is highly motivating and it can bring out the best in a person. As a parent, I think it can help you find out how your child learns best, because it gives you so many exciting avenues to explore. It's a feel-good thing, plus it's a focus for the whole world these days."

In the Workplace

Federal laws protect the rights of employees with disabilities; however, the existence of these laws may not necessarily mean that the supports and services you need will be present in your workplace. It may be up to you, the employee, to educate your employers about what you need to do your job. A simple reacher or grabber might allow you to more safely take cans off a high shelf in a grocery store or pick things up off the floor. A closed-circuit television in a library might help you see to read and write. A computer equipped with specialized software or an adapted keyboard might give you access to print materials, books, or other materials used by the organization where you are working. If you work for a small company, your employer may be unable to afford the accommodations you need. Rather than say, "I can't do that job because I have a disability," ask, "What type of assistive technology is available that will help me do this job?"

At Home and in the Community

We engage in many different types of activities at home, in the community, and as part of daily living. These activities might include going fishing, washing laundry, cooking, grooming ourselves, visiting a local library, participating in clubs or community groups, or going out to eat. As you develop your goals and plans for incorporating assistive technology into your daily routines, ask yourself once again, "What do I want to be able to do? Might assistive technology help me to do it independently?"

> *Khalil*, an elderly man who had a significant hearing loss, wanted to be able to talk on the telephone. An adapted phone with a volume control and a flashing light that announces incoming calls now enables him to hear friends and family when they phone.

Consider every aspect of your life as you make plans for using assistive technology to reach your dreams and goals. Regardless of whether you were born with a disability or acquired a disability through accident, illness, or aging, assistive-technology devices may increase your opportunities and self-sufficiency and contribute to a greater quality of life.

Worksheet 1A: Tracking My AT Plan

Adapted by permission from Bridgett Perry.

Use this worksheet to record information you get and ideas you have while reading through the chapters in Part I. It will help you summarize your progress.

Chapter 1: Creating a Vision

What life situations apply to me?

education _____

_____

_____

transition _____

_____

_____

workplace _____

_____

_____

home _____

_____

_____

community _____

_____

_____

illness/injury _____

_____

_____

aging _____

_____

_____

Worksheet 1A: Tracking My AT Plan (cont'd.)

22

Computer
Resources
for People
with
Disabilities

Description of my vision:

What do I want to be able to do or accomplish (e.g., become a teacher, communicate with my family and friends, live independently)?

_____

_____

_____

What part of this vision may be most difficult or challenging for me?

_____

_____

_____

What interests me, motivates me?

_____

_____

_____

_____

Chapter 2: Achieving My Goals

What specific steps will help me to accomplish the various parts of my vision?

_____

_____

_____

Might any of these tasks be accomplished through technology solutions? Which ones?

_____

_____

_____

Chapter 3: Mobilizing My Resources

Who will help me learn about technology?

_____

_____

Who will help me maintain or care for my technology?

_____

_____

How does my life situation impact the support and resources I need?

_____

_____

_____

Chapter 4: Selecting Technology

Where do I need to use the technology (what environments)?

_____

_____

How effectively can I see a computer screen?

_____

_____

How effectively can I use a keyboard?

_____

_____

How effectively can I use a mouse?

_____

_____

Worksheet 1A: Tracking My AT Plan (cont'd.)

How effectively can I interact with information?

_____

_____

How effectively can I read (comprehend)?

_____

_____

How effectively can I write (compose)?

_____

_____

How effectively can I handle computer equipment?

_____

_____

What are my processing skills in terms of:

Cognitive demands (performing a sequence of commands, using intuitive skills to know what to do next, comprehending prompts or choices offered by the program)?

_____

_____

Academic demands (reading level, spelling, math level, etc.)?

_____

_____

Chapter 5: The Law

Are there laws that protect my rights to assistive technology? What are they?

_____

_____

Whom can I turn to for information about the law and my rights?

_____

_____

What questions do I need to ask?

_____

_____

_____

Chapter 6: Funding Strategies

Are there funding resources to assist me? What are they?

_____

_____

Where can I go and whom can I turn to for information?

_____

_____

What questions do I need to ask?

_____

_____

_____

Chapter 7: Budgeting and Buying

Have I worked out a budget?

_____

Where will I shop?

_____

_____

Worksheet 1A: Tracking My AT Plan (cont'd.)

26

Computer
Resources
for People
with
Disabilities

What questions do I need to ask?

_____

_____

_____

Chapter 8: Up and Running

Do I know where I will set up my equipment?

_____

_____

Do I know where to get help with setting up or troubleshooting my equipment?

_____

_____

Do I need training? If so, who will provide it for me?

_____

_____

Chapter 9: Repairs and Upgrades

What are my upgrade or repair needs?

_____

_____

What choices do I need to make between repairing, upgrading, or replacing my equipment or software?

_____

_____

_____

Chapter 2

Achieving My Goals

How Will Technology Help?

Amy G. Dell, director, Center for Assistive Technology and Inclusive Education Studies at the College of New Jersey, Ewing, New Jersey

Deborah Newton, assistant professor, Center for Assistive Technology and Inclusive Education Studies at the College of New Jersey, Ewing, New Jersey

The Big Picture: Where You Are in Your AT Planning Process

In this chapter we focus on how assistive technology can help you realize your personal vision. At the end of Chapter 1 you were asked to write down your personal vision to serve as sort of a map on your journey to incorporating assistive technology into your life. As you face the many decisions that will need to be made along the way, you can refer back to your vision for guidance and encouragement.

Useful Preparation

At this early stage in the technology search you probably have far more questions now than you had initially. This is a good thing.

- Review the personal vision you developed after reading Chapter 1.

- Think about the key questions you now have or still have after developing your vision.

Steps to Consider

Start by answering the questions in the sections below.

What specifically do I want to be able to do with technology?

"Using a computer" is not a goal in and of itself, but rather a way to achieve other goals. The best decisions about technology are made within the context of a broader vision. Once you have identified your vision (see Chapter 1), you can begin identifying the technology tools that will help you achieve your vision.

What kinds of activities/tasks will my vision require?

You will need to break down your vision into a list of specific activities or tasks that it may entail. For example, if your vision is to attend college, then you need to ask questions like the following: "What specific steps are involved in applying for college? What specific activities/tasks does college-level academic work require?"

Let's continue with the example of attending college. Find a few currently enrolled college students (or recent graduates) and discuss your questions with them. A quick brainstorming session will reveal several essential tasks that all college students need to be able to do:

- read (e.g., textbooks, literature, journal articles, reference books, Internet sites)

- organize one's thoughts

- write: compose and express thoughts clearly

- write: take notes in class and in the library

- conduct research (look for and find relevant information)

- use a computer for research and writing

- attend and listen to lectures and discussions

- manage time and be responsible (e.g., turn in assignments on time)

After the list of required tasks is developed, the next step is to consider the following questions:

Which of these tasks may pose difficulty for me?

For example, if you have a visual impairment, then the tasks that might present a barrier to success may be reading, taking notes, researching information, and using a computer. If you are hard of hearing, then the major barriers may be listening and taking notes in class. If you have a learning disability or attention deficits, then all of these tasks may pose difficulty and require some kind of accommodation.

How can technology help me accomplish these potentially difficult tasks?

Chapter 4 ("Selecting Technology: What's Best for Me?") and Part II ("The Technology Toolbox") provide technical information to help you answer this question. At this point in the process, however, it is helpful to gain a general understanding of how technology can assist with these tasks. Here are some potential technology solutions for several of the specific tasks listed above:

Reading — If you have a visual impairment, a closed-circuit TV (CCTV), also known as a *video magnifier,* can be used to enlarge the print and pictures in any kind of book or printed material. Video magnifiers do this by capturing the text with a small camera and displaying the magnified text on a monitor. These devices come in all sizes—from portable ones that can be carried to different locations, to 21-inch monitors that can display a great deal of text at one time. Some models mount the camera on a swivel head so that the user can turn it towards the blackboard to magnify class notes.

If you are blind and cannot read text of any size, a different solution is available. *Scan/read programs* can read aloud textbooks, journal articles, and class handouts—in short, any kind of printed material. The material is first scanned into a computer using a typical flatbed scanner (which is similar to a copy machine); the computer then translates the text into an electronic format; and the software reads aloud the entire document, at a speed chosen by the reader.

Scan/read programs also offer a powerful technology solution to students with learning disabilities who struggle with reading comprehension and/or slow rates of reading. In addition to reading the text aloud, scan/read programs highlight the text being read and enable you to alter the visual display of the printed material. You can then adjust the appearance so that it is easier to read. For example, you can increase the size of the print, increase the space between lines from single spacing to double spacing (or more), and choose a different background color for contrast. Scan/read programs offer a number of other features that are helpful if you have learning disabilities, including talking dictionaries and the ability to take notes using electronic "highlighters."

Andy is a college graduate who is working in the business world after majoring in marketing. His fourth-grade teacher would be very surprised to learn about his achievements. In fourth grade Andy could not read; in addition, he had poor fine motor skills, low mathematical reasoning, and poor spelling skills, and he was placed in self-contained special education classes. How did he get from being a nonreader to being a successful college graduate? Andy credits his strong motivation, hard work, and his discovery of scan/read technology. In his own words:

The Kurzweil 3000 scan/read program made a huge difference. I literally had 700 pages of retail management, 980 pages of market research, 650 pages of consumer behavior, and 2,000 pages of economic statistics to read. Reading with the Kurzweil 3000 made it easier for me to digest the information. It made a real difference in my comprehension. If I were to read a book like *Marketing Principles* and persevere through all the reading, it would probably take me two and a half hours to read one chapter. By the time I finished reading the last page of the chapter, I would have forgotten the first part of the chapter and would have remembered maybe 40 percent of the rest. Using the scan/read system, it would take me half that time to read the chapter, and I would remember 75–80 percent.

Organizing Thoughts— If you find it difficult to get started with the writing process and are easily overwhelmed by too much information, then you might benefit from software programs that can facilitate the process of getting organized to write. Graphic organizers and outlining programs are easy to use and provide visual guides for brainstorming and organizing ideas. After you enter your ideas onto a concept map and arrange them into a reasonable order, the software—with a single mouse click—will convert the visual map into a text outline. You can then expand the outline into an organized paper using a word processing program.

Writing (Composing) — Many people today prefer writing on a computer using word processing software, as opposed to typing on a typewriter or writing by hand. Why? Because they like the ease of making corrections, of "cutting and pasting" text without having to retype it, and of having their spelling errors caught by a spell checker. If you have a disability, this use of computers may be indispensable. It is a huge time-saver, and the end product has a professional appearance.

Adding specialized software can facilitate the writing process even further. Talking word processing programs, for example, speak aloud everything a person has typed. If you have weak reading skills, you can hear what you've written, rather than what you think you wrote. People with learning disabilities find this to be an essential tool for editing their written work. They also like the fact that the spell checkers in talking word processing programs read aloud misspellings, proper spellings, and dictionary definitions. Some talking word processing programs also include a homonym finder for people who confuse the spellings of words that sound alike (e.g., *to*, *two*, and *too*).

Another kind of software that assists with writing is called *word prediction*. Word prediction programs make an educated guess about the word you are about to type and provide a list of possibilities. You simply select the word you had in mind, and it is then entered into the document. Word prediction offers two main advantages: It speeds up the typing process for people with physical disabilities by reducing the number of keystrokes needed and assists people who have severe spelling problems by providing a word list from which to choose. Most word prediction programs will read aloud the choices presented so a user can choose the correct word after hearing it.

Writing (Taking Notes) — Note taking is listed separately because it is a unique form of writing. By definition, taking notes in class and in the library needs to be a quick process. Any equipment used must be portable enough to be carried from building to building and must last the entire day. Equipment containing a battery that must be charged after a couple of hours has only limited use for note taking in a college environment. For these reasons, laptop computers are often not the best choice for note taking. Handheld personal digital assistants (PDAs) and lightweight note takers offer more portability and less weight; they are also less power hungry. For students who are blind, there are now PDAs available that use a Braille keyboard and provide speech feedback. For students whose note taking is hampered by poor penmanship, portable note takers offer a regular keyboard for in-class use and the ability to connect to a computer for editing later on.

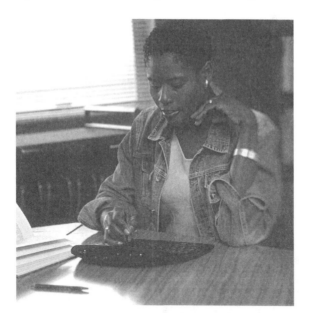

This woman is using the AlphaSmart note taker.
(Photo courtesy of AlphaSmart)

Using a Computer for Research and Writing — Nowadays every college student needs to be able to use a computer. Most college library systems are completely computer-based; registration and campus communication systems rely on computers; term papers are researched and written on computers. Therefore, for students who are unable to use a standard keyboard or see a typical monitor, finding an effective access method is a top priority. Chapter 4 and Part II of this book discuss specific access methods in detail, but this section will provide examples so that the reader can begin to see the possibilities.

If you are a student with visual impairments, you may be able to see the computer screen if all of the print is enlarged. Screen magnification software offers this option. If you lack enough useable vision to read a computer monitor, you will want to look into screen reading programs. These programs read aloud everything on the screen—text, web pages, e-mail messages, menus, submenus, icons, dialogue boxes, etc. These two kinds of assistive technology may make computers accessible to you, enabling you to use computers for research and writing.

If you have a neuromuscular condition like muscular dystrophy, you may lack the strength or range of motion to use a standard keyboard. But one-handed keyboards and mini-keyboards are available that place all the keys much closer together and require less pressure to type. If you have cerebral palsy, you may face a different motor issue: You may be able to reach and press the keys on a regular keyboard, but you might find yourself hitting extra keys. In this situation a keyguard placed over the standard keyboard, combined with turning off the "key repeat" feature in the computer's control panel, may improve your typing significantly. Adding a word prediction program (see "Writing (Composing)," above) will reduce the number of keystrokes needed and increase the rate of typing as well.

Listening — Many hours in college are spent sitting in a classroom, listening and paying attention to professors' lectures. What if you cannot hear well? Deaf students who use sign language usually prefer a sign-language inter-

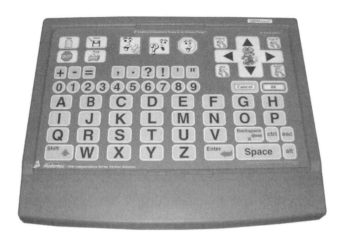

Discover:Board is an alternate keyboard that works like a standard keyboard and mouse. (Photo courtesy of Don Johnston, Inc.)

preter, but if you are hard of hearing and do not sign you may need technology to be able to hear the lecture. Assistive-listening systems are a practical solution. The instructor wears a small microphone and wireless transmitter, and the student wears a small wireless receiver and headphones (or the system can connect directly to a hearing aid). In this way, the instructor's voice is amplified without amplifying all the distracting background noise. Sound-field systems use a similar technology to amplify a teacher's voice for an entire classroom; research suggests that this helps all students pay attention.

Managing Time and Being Responsible — Time management is a major issue for all college students, but it can be particularly troublesome if you have a learning disability, attention deficits, or mental-health issues. Personal digital assistants (PDAs), which have been widely adopted in the corporate world, are now recognized as offering a practical solution to the problems of organization and time management faced by college students with disabilities. The PDA can be set to send reminders to you about important appointments and deadlines. Software is available that enables you to enter all assignment deadlines on both your "to-do lists" and calendars, while linking those notes to the actual assignments. It is important to note that if you lack personal organization and time-management skills, you will need to be *taught* how to make the most of these technology tools.

How Life Situations Impact Achieving Your Goals with Assistive Technology

Preschool Through Primary Grades

Parents' visions for their young children often focus on their being able to participate in play activities and socialize with other children. At first it may not be obvious how technology can help achieve these goals. However, a group of parents, teachers, and assistive-technology companies have been working for many years on developing products to facilitate these types of activities. At a technology-access center in Berkeley, California, for example, parents brought their children to "technology playgroups" with the goal of developing social skills and having fun with their friends. Of course they also learned important skills. With battery-operated cars attached to large, brightly colored switches, they developed switch skills that they could later use to operate computers. By attaching marking pens to the toy cars, running them over huge sheets of butcher paper, and watching them crash into each other, they experienced the joy of creating "art" and playing together.

In your search for ideas and solutions, be sure to consider "low-tech" approaches, especially with children. They are usually low-cost and readily available. Often, low-tech AT is most like that used by typical peers. Low-tech solutions can help you determine if it is wise to invest in a more expensive, commercially available alternative in the future. Additionally, low-tech solutions are often easier to use; they take much less know-how, and you may be more comfortable using them or supporting their use.

Low-tech solutions have two limitations that you need to consider. Because they are simple and unsophisticated, they often address only one specific issue, and they may have limited capacity to keep pace with changing needs due to a child's growth and development or changes in physical abilities.

You may find the following low-tech ideas helpful for children in this age group:

Recreation

- Attach wooden knobs sold at craft and hobby stores to toys such as miniature cars and trucks or to puzzle pieces to make them easier to grasp.

- Fill a small plastic tray with about one inch of plaster of Paris. Insert the cap end of colored markers into the plaster and let it harden. Users can now independently select, use, and recap markers.

- Put toys or other objects on a solid black or yellow vinyl place mat or tablecloth to increase visual contrast.

- Put Velcro on the thumb and palm of a knit glove or mitten and on the exterior of crayons, markers, toys, and other items to assist those with a limited grasp.

- Use permanent markers on a cookie sheet to draw a tic-tac-toe grid or other game board. Put magnets on the back of playing pieces so they will adhere to the board. Use playing pieces that are big enough to grasp, such as empty film canisters. Wrap canisters with colorful tape in two different colors to signify the X and the O pieces, or place brightly colored sticker dots on the lids.

- Use a hairbrush as a cardholder to enable participation in card games. Velcro the hairbrush to a nonskid place mat if necessary.

- Use Rubbermaid or Contact nonslip shelf liner to keep arts-and-craft projects, as well as other items, from sliding away.

Reading and Writing

- Use a plate display stand to hold papers in an upright position for easy viewing.

- To reduce glare from materials printed on white paper, place papers in a transparent, colored file holder.

- Eliminate visual distractions and help with visual tracking by making a reading guide. Cut a rectangular opening in a strip of poster board. The opening should be cut to match the length and height of the lines of text to be read. Cover the board with clear Contact paper to increase its durability. A similar construction can also be used as a handwriting guide. Cut the opening to about the size that you want the largest letters to be, and write within the opening.

- Use a three-inch or five-inch ring binder as a slant board. Use binder clips to keep papers in place.

- Turn lined paper sideways to help with lining up numbers when writing math problems.

- Place pens or pencils inside foam hair rollers to make them easier to grasp.

Communication

- Cut pictures from grocery-store and department-store sale circulars to create communication boards. Cover the communication boards with clear Contact paper to increase their durability.

- Attach small pieces of self-adhesive magnetic tape to the backs of picture/symbol cards. Place cards on a cookie sheet, refrigerator door, or any magnetic surface to create instant communication boards.

- Use dry-erase Contact paper to create "write on, wipe off" communication boards. Attach a dry-erase marker so that it is readily available.

- Use a clear cosmetic bag to hold a variety of small boards that will be easy to carry.

James's story illustrates how "simple technology" can be used in school settings to facilitate socialization and play. James was a six-year-old boy with cerebral palsy. His parents' ultimate goal for him was inclusion in a regular primary class. An early step toward this goal was adapting the childhood game red light/green light so that he could participate. Using two simple *talking switches,* one red and one green, James made his selection by pressing one of them, and it would say either "red light" or "green light." The class, assembled in a circle, responded to James' commands by walking or stopping, as appropriate. (In the traditional game, students line up and try to reach the finish line first. The switch version was designed to be noncompetitive so students of all abilities could enjoy it.) The simple game soon had everyone laughing, and James was thrilled. The computer had empowered him as a leader. Red light/green light was particularly successful for James because it was something he really enjoyed doing, it made technology part of the curriculum rather than a separate activity, and there were no wrong answers since the class responded to whatever choice James made.

Education: K–12

At the beginning of this chapter we discussed breaking down your vision into a list of activities that it may entail, and we used the example of attending college. If your vision for your school-aged child includes having him or her be an active participant in his or her education, then you need to brainstorm about the typical activities that take place in classrooms.

Ask yourself this question: What kinds of activities/tasks regularly take place in my child's classroom or school? Some of your answers will be the same as for college-level work (for example, writing), but many of the details will be different. For example, in elementary schools some of the writing demands relate to completing worksheets. Note taking is rarely an issue in the early grades, but painting and drawing activities are common. Worksheet 2A, starting on the next page, will help you identify the specific educational activities for which you would like to find technology solutions. (The worksheet is written in the first person, but if you're completing it on behalf of your child, of course, the questions should be answered from his or her perspective.) Chapter 4 and Part II will help you pinpoint specific products to explore.

Worksheet 2A: Prioritizing My Activities

My vision (write it here):

_____

_____

_____

Questions to ponder:

Which of the following tasks or activities are my priorities? (Check all that apply.)	Which are difficult for me?
☐ **Writing:**	☐
☐ handwriting (problems with pen and paper)	☐
☐ completing worksheets ("seatwork")	☐
☐ composition: story writing	☐
☐ composition: journal writing	☐
☐ encouragement/motivation to write	☐
☐ prewriting activities (organizing thoughts, outlining)	☐
☐ note taking	☐
☐ spelling	☐
☐ Reading:	☐
☐ reading instruction	☐
☐ increasing comprehension of content	☐
☐ finding high-interest/low-level reading materials	☐
☐ being able to see the reading materials	☐
☐ converting reading materials to Braille	☐
☐ **Research ("looking up" information for a report or project)**	☐
☐ **Calculating (addition, subtraction, multiplication, etc.)**	☐

Worksheet 2A: Prioritizing My Activities (cont'd.)

Which of the following tasks or activities are my priorities? (Check all that apply.)	Which are difficult for me?
☐ **Practicing academic skills (e.g., multiplication tables, spelling words)**	☐
☐ **Artistic expression:**	☐
☐ painting, drawing	☐
☐ theatrics	☐
☐ music	☐
☐ **Verbal expression**	☐
☐ **Simulating inaccessible or dangerous activities (e.g., software that simulates participation in science experiments involving dissection or dangerous chemicals)**	☐
☐ **Gaining reasoning and higher-level thinking skills**	☐
☐ **Completing homework independently**	☐
☐ **Other:**	☐

_____

_____

_____

_____

_____

In the Workplace

With the advent of the Americans with Disabilities Act (1990), jobs are now described in terms of the *functions* required of an employee. For example, a particular job might require placing and answering telephone calls, accessing a computer database, and preparing written reports. Once these functions have been specified, conventional and assistive technologies can be identified to help with them as needed. Thus, the strategy for achieving an employment vision consists of developing a list of essential job functions and gaining access to those functions using technology.

Nick is an engineer, recently retired from the U.S. Army Corps of Engineers. His job involved monitoring flooding and protecting homes, commerce, and traffic along the river. When he developed multiple sclerosis and became legally blind, keeping the job he loved and remaining productive required him to find some new ways of doing business.

Working with his state department for the blind and later with his local technology-access center, Nick gained access to the computers and software used at his previous position through a combination screen magnification/screen reading program. He needed access to a specific spreadsheet program to monitor readings and perform calculations, and to a word processing program to report findings. With access to the necessary technology, Nick was able to remain a fine engineer and to reach

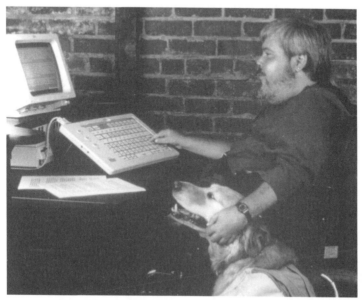

*Adults with disabilities may find programmable keyboards
useful for a variety of purposes—employment, productivity,
communication. (Photo courtesy of IntelliTools)*

retirement with the Corps after nine more years. Following retirement he established an engineering-consulting business in his home.

Shenita is a social worker who needs to type many reports. She is a one-handed typist because of her cerebral palsy. Unfortunately, she developed carpal tunnel syndrome in the hand that she uses to type. Surgery was ruled out for her, so she needed to find another solution. She has found success with an alternate keyboard called IntelliKeys. The angle and the sensitivity of this keyboard allow her to type without pain. She has also added a word prediction program that allows her to type using fewer keystrokes. These accommodations are making it possible for her to continue her work as a social worker and complete the required reports.

At Home/Daily Living

In addition to enabling people to attend school, work in the community, enjoy recreational activities, and socialize, assistive technology can also empower people with disabilities to live more self-sufficiently. An *environmental-control system* can control thermostats and lighting in the home, operate an intercom system and front-door lock, place and receive telephone calls, send out an alert for help, and run a home entertainment system.

Jim sustained a spinal-cord injury over 16 years ago and has gained independence through the use of a sophisticated environmental-control system. Using his computer, he explains how his system works.

> Because of the high level of my injury, I am unable to use my hands and arms in a functional manner. A few years ago I learned of a person who could help me get a voice-operated system to control my environment. He customized my computer system using a voice recognition program and an environmental-control module that allows me to turn lights on and off, answer and originate phone calls, control a television, open and close my garage door, and unlock my back door, all by voice commands. A microphone is mounted on my wheelchair, and so is a speaker, through which I get speech feedback from the system. In this way, I can be anywhere in my home and still use the voice recognition system to control my environment. There is also a microphone and speaker mounted by my bed so that I can respond to any emergency during the night. This particular aspect has given me a much greater peace of mind than I have ever had since my injury. I greatly enjoy the independence I have gained from this environmental-control system.

Other computer applications that can increase self-sufficiency in daily living are shopping and banking online. Many department stores, specialty stores, catalog companies, and banks have websites that enable customers to shop and bank from home at any hour of the day or night. Once you have access to a computer, a world of new resources becomes available to you.

Injury, Illness, and Aging

Remember that the process of identifying technology tools to make an activity or task possible begins with your initial vision. If you are trying to find effective technology as you experience changes in your physical abilities or senses due to an injury, chronic illness, or aging, the process still begins with a vision. What, specifically, do you want to be able to do with technology? If you want to attend college, the example provided at the beginning of this chapter would be applicable; if your vision relates to employment, the examples of Nick and Shenita are instructive. If, however, your priorities focus more on enhancing communication and leisure activities, you will want to read about Sidney.

> *Sidney* has multiple sclerosis and no longer has the ability to control any movement from his neck down. He lives in a nursing home around the corner from the church where he is a visiting minister. The church's members wanted to take up a collection to help Sidney realize more independence. They gave him a choice between a motorized wheelchair and a computer. Sidney chose the computer.
>
> Sidney very much wanted to write to friends around the country and even in town. Before getting his computer, he had to wait for someone to bring him a telephone and hold it for him while he spoke. Now he easily communicates online via e-mail. No more answering machines, busy signals, or waiting for assistance, and he is able to carry on private communications when and how he wishes.
>
> Sidney was an avid reader before his illness, but his multiple sclerosis prevents him from holding a book or turning pages independently. He deeply missed the intellectual stimulation reading offered him. Now, however, with his computer providing access to the Internet, he has access to thousands (millions, if he had the time) of volumes, including the Bible, encyclopedias, and a wide range of resources on great works of art. He can browse through the collections of the Metropolitan Museum of Art in New York or the Louvre in Paris. He also uses his computer to play a variety of games, from Wheel of Fortune to bridge. He feels that the computer has saved his sanity.
>
> Since Sidney cannot move from the neck down, how does he use his computer? He uses a head-mounted mouse emulator called a

HeadMaster, with an on-screen keyboard. He uses a puff switch to replace the mouse click. The on-screen keyboard was set up by Sidney. If he needs a new key, he adds it. The camera key in the middle of the keyboard was added so he can take snapshots of the screen and import the graphics into his letters to his grandchildren.

Technology has afforded Sidney a life of intellectual stimulation, despite his living in a nursing home, and a level of independence that he thought he would never retrieve.

The example of Sidney illustrates the many possibilities offered by computer technology for hobbies, entertainment, and other forms of recreation. Thousands of popular games, such as poker, chess, television game shows, and board games, have been adapted for computers, providing people with disabilities access to games that otherwise would be inaccessible. Thousands more adventure games and simulations have been designed specifically for computers. Many Internet services and websites enable users to compete online with fellow gaming enthusiasts in other locations, including overseas.

Virtually every hobby or interest can be explored and enhanced via the millions of individuals and businesses now using the Internet. Would you like to find specialized tools for gardening and to meet other gardeners who use wheelchairs? Would you like to know where the accessible fishing sites or nature trails are located in your state? Would you like to explore archives of photographs and the memories of specific individuals in order to put together a multimedia presentation for an upcoming special event? Are you a "Star Trek" fan? Do you enjoy comic books? Would you like to shop for magic tricks or for the equipment you might need to try your hand at making home-brewed beer? All these hobbies and countless more can be discovered and explored on the Internet.

Communication

Being able to express one's thoughts, feelings, and ideas is absolutely critical to being successful in school, the workplace, recreational settings, and the community. Being able to understand other people's communication attempts is equally essential. If you are a person who cannot speak or who cannot hear speech, technology offers an exciting range of solutions. If you have difficulty articulating speech clearly, assistive technology can literally provide a voice. *Augmentative* or *alternative communication* (*AAC* or *augcomm*, for short) systems range widely in size, complexity, and price, but what all technology-based systems have in common is a method to store communication messages and the use of speech output to express them.

If finding an effective augmentative communication system is part of your vision, we recommend that you seek a qualified speech/language specialist who has experience in augmentative communication technology to assist you in selecting the right solution. Together, you will consider many important factors, such as fine motor skills, language and cognitive abilities, vocabulary needs, environments in which the augcomm system will be needed, portability needs, the kind of training and technical support needed, and room for growth. After these factors have been explored, the specialist can help you select the system that best matches your specific needs.

Anthony is a young man who works for an augmentative-communication business. He has cerebral palsy, which has interfered with his ability to speak, and he has become an expert on, and an advocate for, augcomm systems. Anthony has advice for parents and professionals:

> One of the things I like to emphasize is that communication development doesn't just happen overnight, which is a common assumption made by parents, teachers, and therapists. I received my first communication board with six pictures on it at the age of two. By the time I reached elementary school I had a board with almost 100 symbols on it. When there was no more room to put words on the board, my parents and therapists started researching other methods. That's when they found one of the first computer-based augmentative communication systems in 1984. When I

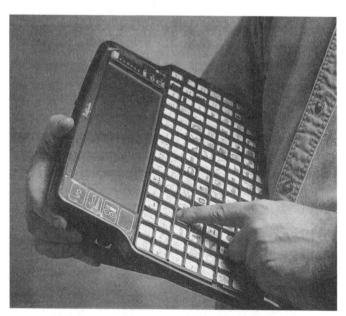

*This man can converse using an augmentative
communication device from Prentke Romich.
(Photo courtesy of Prentke Romich Company)*

received my TouchTalker, it was the happiest day of my childhood. My augcomm device enabled me to attend public school and fully participate in all school activities.

Later I began working for an augmentative-communication company as an ambassador, traveling to conferences to display the powers of my system (my second computer-based augcomm device). Today, using my latest augcomm system, the Pathfinder, I work as a remote troubleshooter for the company. I answer technical service calls about the company's products at night and on weekends when the company is closed. Without a doubt, I would be unable to be employed at a meaningful job if I did not have access to my augmentative communication device.

If you are deaf or hard of hearing, you may not hear well enough to use a standard telephone, so adaptations or alternatives are needed to be able to communicate with people over distances. Amplified phones allow users to adjust the volume and control the tone, similar to boosting the bass on your stereo. Telecommunication devices for the deaf (TDD, also known as TTYs), which are equipped with a keyboard and small visual display, enable users to type messages and send them over the phone lines. With the proliferation of cell phones, you can take advantage of text-messaging capabilities in cell-phone plans. Text messaging offers a new level of convenience and liberation since users no longer have to be tied to a TTY.

● ● ●

We hope this chapter has helped you begin to explore the possibilities of using assistive technology to enrich your life.

Chapter 3

Mobilizing My Resources

Where Do I Start?

Perrine Dailey, assistive-technology specialist, PACER Simon Technology Center, Minneapolis, Minnesota

Marcia J. Scherer, Ph.D., Director, Institute for Matching Person and Technology, Webster, New York

The Big Picture: Where You Are in Your AT Planning Process

It is not always easy to know where to begin, who to talk to, or what questions to ask when starting the process of obtaining appropriate technology. This chapter will guide you through the steps involved in finding resources, support, and knowledge. It focuses on helping you build a circle of supportive people to aid your search. Having that resource in place will boost your confidence and empower you to communicate your needs and capabilities—in other words, to self-advocate. *Self-advocacy* means doing for yourself by gathering the information and support to make decisions and choices on your own, rather than relying on other people to make them for you.

Useful Preparation

As you begin, keep in mind your vision of how technology can help you and the plan you've developed to assist you in achieving that vision.

- If you do not yet have a vision, read Chapter 1, "Creating a Vision: Why Do I Need A Plan?"

- If you are unsure about how assistive-technology devices can help you, refer to Chapter 2, "Achieving My Goals: How Will Technology Help?"

- Don't panic about how to pay for the devices. There is lots of useful information about funding resources in Chapter 6, "Funding Strategies: How Will I Pay for It All?"

Steps to Consider

Building Your Circle of Support

When you are just beginning the search for assistive technology, it is common to feel isolated, scared, and intimidated by the process ahead. Having a circle of support will be a welcome comfort. It will also offer a pool of talent and knowledge to draw on for questions or assistance, even while you retain control over the process and decisions.

Keep the following suggestions in mind when building your circle of support:

- **Turn first to those closest to you.** The people who already support you probably know you well enough to offer sound advice. They can help you consider all the areas in which you might benefit from using technology.

- **Consider including family, friends, neighbors, and coworkers who see you on a regular basis.** These individuals will eventually interact with the technology that you select, including making accommodations once the technology is actively being used. Someone familiar with the environment in which you plan to use your technology may also be very helpful.

- **Include a professional with relevant expertise.** Doing so may be especially important if you anticipate the need for customized equipment. For example, a speech pathologist may be of help if you need a communication system.

- **Consider including a trained advocate.** An advocate can help if you are concerned about your rights under the law or about challenges from a potential source of funding.

- **Keep your goals in mind as you build a circle of support.** Refer back to Chapter 2 for more information on goal setting. Think about who you are, what you need, and why. With this awareness you can more easily and effectively communicate your needs to your team, and your team will be better equipped to help you make the right technology choices.

- **Consider the people you've already met who have knowledge about assistive technology.** For example:

  - What computers or assistive devices, if any, are you using now? How are you using them? Who was most helpful to you in getting them and learning to use them?

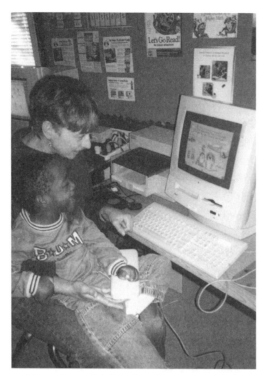

*Through a guided exploration process, many
people find their technology solutions at a
local Alliance Center. (Photo courtesy of
Carolina Computer Access Center)*

— If you're considering a new type of technology, have you seen anyone use it? Can you contact that person to learn more about the
product?

— Is there anyone in your social network, workplace, or community
who knows about assistive technologies? Contact them for
support.

Pedro is a kindergartner with Down syndrome. Pedro's family members
had become accustomed to his inability to express himself with words.
They relied on "mind reading" to provide Pedro with what he wanted.
When a new piece of assistive technology in the form of an augmentative
communication device was introduced to Pedro, the whole family
needed to adapt to the change. The new device provided the tools Pedro
needed to communicate. However, to use it successfully, he needed his
family members to actively use it with him and offer him multiple communication opportunities throughout the day instead of continuing to
"mind read."

Before the device was available, Pedro had never been asked to choose what kind of snack he preferred. Instead, his parents would make the decision for him. Now, his parents can give him a choice and allow him the time he needs to make his decision and express it to them.

Jeffrey, a first-year college student with low vision, is beginning to feel frustrated with the amount of time he spends doing course work. Because he chose to attend a college away from home, he no longer has easy access to many members of his circle of support, such as his parents, siblings, high-school teachers, and friends.

Jeffrey has 20/200 uncorrected vision, 20/80 corrected vision, and impaired peripheral vision. He lives on campus, where he uses various low-tech, portable, commercially available devices that offer him mobility without being obtrusive. He has not yet used more sophisticated technologies and does not know Braille. He places a high priority on avoiding standing out in his classes and among his peers. He does, however, use a cane for safety and mobility.

Jeffrey was unaware of the existence of his college's Disability Support Office. He feels that most technologies available to students on campus are either in disrepair or inaccessible to him due to their location and inconvenience. Thus far in his college career, Jeffrey has not identified himself as a student in need of support.

Because Jeffrey is only a freshman and both college life and the campus are new to him, he could benefit by adding a person from the Disability Support Office to his local circle of support. This person could offer Jeffrey assistance in finding such services as help with note taking, classroom and testing accommodations, and alternate ways of accomplishing tasks without attracting attention to himself. Building a comfort level with college life also includes exploring social participation on campus. As Jeffrey develops a sense of belonging and further expands his circle of support, he may grow to feel more comfortable about using new assistive technologies that he currently fears will separate him from his peers.

Bearing in mind the issues addressed in this chapter, think about who you would like to include in your circle of support. Also think about *how* you would like for each supporter to be involved. Then list their names below. Include both those you already know will "be there" for you (e.g., your spouse) and those you may need to approach about being on your team (e.g., your next-door neighbor who's a computer expert).

Note that this list is dynamic rather than static. It is very likely that you will add names to it in the coming days, weeks, and months as you continue to learn about resources and gather information.

Myself	
Relatives	**Neighbors**
Friends	**Community organizations**
College/high-school contacts	**Religious organizations**
Colleagues at work	**Therapists**
Teachers	**Hospitals/Agencies**

Finding Resources and Support

You may be surprised to discover how many resources are available where you can learn more about assistive technology, no matter what your situation. Take advantage of these sources of information. Even if a particular source doesn't sound useful to you, don't ignore it; it may be able to refer you to other, more useful sources.

What follows is a list of resources to get you started. Some agencies are staffed by highly trained professionals and are extremely well equipped with assistive devices, software, and hardware; others have yet to discover technology. With perseverance you will uncover the most useful resources in your own community.

After each conversation or meeting, use a blank sheet formatted like the example below to record the information you collected. Include the name and phone number of other contacts you may have obtained, as well as any specific plans for following up or pursuing other strategies. Then consider whether any of the individuals you've made contact with are candidates for inclusion in the list of supportive people you compiled in Worksheet 3A.

Sample Contact Record

Date	Phone #	Contact name and address	What happened? / Ideas for follow-up
4/7/04	800-53PACER	PACER Center Simon Technology Center	Has many resources. Plan a tour; check future workshops.

Assistive-technology centers and community technology centers (CTCs)

These offer a wide variety of resources. Call, write, or visit a center if there is one in your community. There are many types of assistive-technology centers. Many belong to the Alliance for Technology Access (ATA). The staff and volunteers at ATA centers provide hands-on opportunities to explore assistive technology in an environment free of architectural and attitudinal barriers. There are no eligibility requirements, and everyone seeking assistance is served, regardless of age or type of disability. Alliance centers take an approach that places the potential user at the hub of the process as the evaluator of the equipment and software, rather than as the object of evaluation. The centers are committed to helping you develop the expertise you need to make the best decisions.

Alliance centers offer comprehensive, multifaceted programs that reflect community needs and local talents and resources. Although each center is unique, all of them provide services that help children and adults with disabilities, parents, teachers, and employers explore computer systems, adaptive devices, and software. Once you are connected to an Alliance center, you are in touch with a large network of individuals with disabilities, parents, educators, friends, and vendors who are glad to share their expertise.

Besides ATA centers, assistive-technology centers can often be found at colleges and universities, local chapters of disability-specific organizations, independent-living centers, community centers, churches, and other places. A little research within your community may net you a great resource in your search for technology solutions.

Independent-living centers (ILCs)

ILCs and other consumer groups that are led primarily by adults with disabilities are another excellent resource. ILCs exist primarily to support individuals with disabilities in reaching self-defined goals. The level of knowledge about assistive technologies varies greatly among centers, but many have valuable resources to share. ILCs are open to any adult with a disability; other consumer groups may serve individuals with specific disabilities. Since they are community-based programs, they reflect the needs and resources of the individual community.

Your state's department of vocational rehabilitation

It may offer assistive technology or training as part of its job-placement program. The staff may also be able to point you to other local resources. (The office may go by a different name in your state, such as the Department of Rehabilitation Services or the Department of Rehabilitation.)

College and university disability services

These offices are dedicated to coordinating services for students with disabilities and to providing access to college life through self-advocacy, accommodations, and technology. Facilities and expertise may be located on campus, or you may be referred to local community resources such as an ILC. These programs address a wide range of issues, including housing, transportation, physical access to facilities, and curriculum adaptations, to name a few. They may or may not be thoroughly knowledgeable about assistive technology. However, with so many legislative mandates in place, colleges and universities are moving closer with each passing year to becoming models of access.

Public schools

Under the law, public schools must provide disabled infants, toddlers, children, youth, and young adults a free public education, up to the age of 22. Every public school system in the United States has a special-education department or some cooperative arrangement for providing special education and related services. You may find teachers, therapists, or other individuals in the special-education department who have expertise to share. You may also find educators who are well versed in technology and able to provide assistance.

A school system will often have an individual on staff who coordinates assistive-technology resources for the entire district. Although these individuals may be busy and difficult to find, the effort may be worthwhile as they can often provide valuable information. You may be able to schedule time to explore the district's equipment and to observe students using it. Call the special-education department to identify the people on staff who are most knowledgeable in assistive technologies.

Parent groups

These provide information and support to family members of children with disabilities. The types and strengths of parent groups vary greatly. In the mid-1970s, a federal program to establish a national network of community-based parent training and information (PTI) centers was created. These centers inform parents of their child's educational rights and assist them in their advocacy efforts. Parents and family members are always welcome to join an environment in which they can share and contribute from their own experience. Some of these centers are good resources for assistive technology.

Disability agencies

Agencies serving children and adults with disabilities can be private for-profit or not-for-profit organizations, such as Easter Seals, United Cerebral Palsy, and The Arc (formerly Association for Retarded Citizens). Some may provide opportunities for hands-on computer demonstrations and explorations. Disability agencies usually have restrictions regarding whom they can serve, which may vary by age, disability, and geographic area. However, although they may not usually serve people with your disability or zip code, they may be happy to discuss or share with you the assistive technologies they are using or refer you to other resources.

Many disability organizations operate technology projects under grants from the government or from private foundations. For example, the federally funded Family Center on Technology and Disability is focused on providing technology information to organizations serving families of children and youth with disabilities.

Disability newspapers and newsletters

These contain both articles and advertisements that may offer valuable information. Many disability newspapers print regular features on conventional and assistive technologies or announcements of meetings and events that can help in your networking efforts.

Vendors of assistive technologies

Vendors are a great resource. When you contact some of the resources listed in this section, such as a technology-access center, disability newspaper, special-education department, or independent-living center, you can gather names and addresses of vendors of assistive technologies and services. Vendors can provide you with information about their products and may be able to furnish you with names and phone numbers for additional resources or upcoming events in your area. Most vendors can be contacted through their websites and e-mail addresses.

The Internet

An abundance of information about assistive technology can be found on the Internet. Most assistive-technology vendors have comprehensive websites that show images of their products and list features and prices. Many non-profit organizations operate websites that offer a wealth of information about assistive technology. You can also use a search engine to locate products and even download demonstration software. Simply type in the name or type of product and browse the sites. The more specific you can be about the product, such as knowing the name of the product or vendor, the more useful information you will find.

The Internet is also a great source of information about the laws pertaining to assistive technology. Many resources are available that can provide you with the text of laws, legislative updates, and alerts, as well as information about advocacy efforts taking place.

A growing number of online computer services sponsor forums focused on the use of technology by people with disabilities. The individuals who participate in these forums and who use online bulletin-board services can provide up-to-date information.

Medical professionals

Doctors, nurses, occupational and physical therapists, psychiatrists, psychologists, and so on, can be good resources. Ask them to refer you to helpful resources, including current articles in medical journals or new research they may know about.

Teachers' colleges and university schools of education

These programs train educators. Programs for special education and related services often have a faculty member who is knowledgeable about assistive technology and who may be able to provide you with access to equipment and information resources. You may want to inquire about taking an introductory class in assistive technology.

Libraries

Libraries offer a number of resources that will be useful to you. Libraries stock a wealth of books and periodicals that cover conventional computing, and you will find reference books cataloged under the topic of computers. The reference librarian can suggest current periodicals such as *MacWorld, PC Magazine, T.H.E. Journal* (Technology Horizons in Education), *Electronic Learning,* and *Technology and Learning.* Although they are a bit technical for the novice, these periodicals are still useful sources of new product information. Most of them are also available at local bookstores and computer stores.

Check out the more specialized journals available in colleges and some public libraries that regularly discuss aspects of assistive technology and that can refer you to other sources. Some of these journals are *Closing the Gap, Exceptional Parent Magazine, Journal of Special Education Technology, Journal of Vision Impairment and Blindness,* and *Assistive Technology Journal.* They contain a variety of articles on new products, strategies for using assistive technology in the classroom, resources, and personal stories.

Libraries can also be a good source of information about local organizations, since libraries are often on mailing lists to receive newsletters and brochures. Many libraries also provide free public access to the Internet, and some are beginning to acquire assistive technology to make their computers accessible in compliance with their ADA obligations.

Friends and neighbors

Friends who are computer users can be valuable resources in your search for technology solutions. Friends who use technology at work or at home should be able to advise you about places to shop and things to avoid. They can be enlisted to help you carry boxes, hook up your computer, or make telephone calls. Technology can be so energizing and contagious that you may discover a new friend or two.

One word of caution, however: Friends may be unaware of your specific needs, so make sure the advice you get is compatible with those needs.

User groups

Groups of computer enthusiasts who get together to share new technologies and practical tips may be good contacts. Some groups are so large that they are subdivided into special-interest groups, such as educators, accountants, and dentists. Some groups are dedicated to specific disabilities. User groups are usually focused around a particular type of computer or operating system, such as Windows, Macintosh, or Linux.

The main benefit of connecting with user groups is learning about conventional technologies. For example, if personal financial-management software is of interest to you, a user-group member can probably teach you everything you need to know about the topic. User groups are outstanding places to obtain public-domain software, demonstration programs, and shareware programs. Members of user groups tend to be knowledgeable, helpful, and enthusiastic. What they may lack in assistive-technology experience they will make up for with motivation, commitment to helping others, and ingenuity. Some user groups have even become interested in funding assistive technology.

Computer dealers and stores

Retailers can be a good place to begin learning about conventional technology. Keep in mind that dealers generally have not been exposed at all to the field of assistive technology and will probably be unable to answer your questions related to access and assistive technology, especially if the end user has a moderate to severe disability.

How Life Situations Impact Building a Circle of Support

The resources you utilize will vary according to your particular life situation. Below we list some possible resources for various life stages and circumstances.

Preschool

- Contact the office of early intervention services in your county.

- Familiarize yourself with the benefits your child may be entitled to under the law (see Chapter 5).

- Find other parents who have successfully worked with the same system you are working with; they will have valuable experiences and insights to share with you.

- Learn about organizations in your community that can provide guidance and link you with experienced parents (e.g., the United Cerebral Palsy Associations).

K–12 (Public or Private)

- Contact the state department of education.

- Familiarize yourself with the benefits your child may be entitled to under the law, in particular under IDEA and Section 504 of the Rehabilitation Act (see Chapter 5).

- Find other parents who have successfully worked with the same school system you are working with; they will have valuable experiences and insights to share with you.

- Attend PTA meetings to meet other parents.

Higher Education

- Contact your state division or office of vocational rehabilitation to find information about training opportunities or equipment that may be available to you.

- Visit the campus office of disability support services.

- Familiarize yourself with relevant legislation, including Section 504 of the Rehabilitation Act and the Higher Education Act (see Chapter 5).

- Join campus groups of interest to you.

Transition from School to Work

- Ensure that a transition plan is in place, as required by law (IDEA).

- Check your state's department of rehabilitation and vocation for resources, which may include individuals knowledgeable about job training as well as individuals who are knowledgable about the purchase of assistive technology and about training programs for the use of this technology.

- Get ideas and strategies by talking with other individuals who have completed their transition from school to work.

In the Workplace

- Contact the human-resources department to find experts in reasonable accommodations; people who can open doors to employment.

- Make sure that your supervisor and coworkers are informed about your needs.

- Familiarize yourself with the Americans with Disabilities Act (ADA).

Back to Work (Reentry)

- Contact the county or state vocational rehabilitation services office to locate individuals knowledgeable about job retraining and assistive technology that can make job reentry successful.

- Find self-help groups that may offer useful support.

- When possible, arrange to visit your work site after an illness or injury but before you start back to work. Doing so will allow you to break the ice with your coworkers and ease back into the milieu.

Injury, Illness

- Find out if your community has a loan center for temporary device needs.

- Join a support group for help in determining the accommodations and resources that are most appropriate for you.

Aging

- Contact your local agencies on aging (e.g., office for the aging, senior-citizen center, community education) for information and support.

- Join a support group to gain from other people's experiences.

After contacting a variety of resources, you should have a core group of people you can count on as your circle of support. These are the folks who will be there for you as you continue your process of obtaining assistive technology to help you achieve your goals. Each person in your circle is important and plays a unique role. Contact the people in your circle for encouragement, to share success stories, to exchange information, and to get answers and suggestions.

Now that you have your circle of support in place and are equipped with a knowledge of local resources, you are prepared to select the assistive technology most appropriate for you. The next chapter will lead you through that process.

Chapter 4

Selecting Technology

What Products Are Best for Me?

Lisa Wahl, consultant, Berkeley, California

Kirsten Haugen, assistive-technology and education consultant, Eugene, Oregon

The Big Picture: Where You Are in Your AT Planning Process

In this chapter we focus on the selection process for choosing assistive-technology products. Selecting the right AT is especially critical if you have a one-shot chance at funding. Something may look perfect when demonstrated by a vendor, but if it's too hard to use or doesn't meet your needs, it will sit idle. The following are some steps in the overall process that may directly influence the way you approach this phase:

- **Assess your technology needs and set your goals.** Are you clear about what you want to be able to accomplish with the support of technology? The answers to this question will impact which technology to select. (Refer to Chapter 2 for suggestions on how to assess your needs and set goals.)

- **Determine your "people" resources and build a circle of support.** Have you identified who can help you through the planning process, who else to contact, and how to build a team of support? Doing so may make the process easier when it comes time to select technology that is appropriate for you. (Refer to Chapter 3 for information on tapping into your "people" resources.)

- **Consider your funding strategies.** Which funding strategies could help you pay for the technology? This may impact which technology you can afford to select. (Refer to Chapter 5 for information about the laws and your rights, and to Chapter 6 for information on funding strategies.)

- Use the worksheets in this chapter to organize your selection process. You may wish to make photocopies of them so you can keep track of your progress and take notes.

- Browse the product descriptions in Part II (organized by input, processing, and output) to gain an overview of the variety of technology solutions available.

- Think about the following considerations before making any big purchases.

A Word on Macintosh vs. PC

The computer you use will most likely be running a Windows or Macintosh operating system. Your choice will reflect which one you find easier to use, which is required for the software and assistive technology you need, or perhaps the requirements of your school or work setting. We don't recommend one system over another, because the choice is a personal one and depends on a great many variables. Fans of each system tend to be loyal and vocal in their praise of their particular brand and model. You may want to keep an open mind until you look at the features that are most important to you.

The "Real" Cost of Technology

As part of your planning, consider the cost of software and training. An individual may well spend more on software in the first couple of years of computer ownership than was spent on the computer hardware itself. When comparing systems, be sure to note which software is included and what you'll need to add. For example, most new computers have a word processing program preinstalled, which may be perfect for your writing needs. However, if you want to dictate, rather than type, text into the word processing program, you may spend $200 or more for the voice-input software you will need. And if you are a beginning computer user, you may need a tutor to work with you on any software that has a significant learning curve.

Finally, there is no "best" piece of software—or for that matter, no "best" piece of hardware for someone with a disability—just as there is no best novel or best automobile. Your individual preferences, needs, and resources will determine your software and hardware options, just as they do your choice of books and vehicles.

Old vs. New

The assistive technology you are buying now, or will want to add in the coming year, will be designed to run on the latest computer systems. While a two- to three-year-old computer for $500 may look like a bargain, odds are good that it won't be as satisfactory as something current.

Steps to Consider

The remainder of this chapter will guide you through the details of selecting assistive-technology products. The material is organized with the following questions in mind. (Worksheet 4E, located at the end of the chapter, gives you a chance to reflect on your responses to these questions.)

- What do I need the technology to do?

- What are my strengths and weaknesses?

- What are the settings or environments where the technology will be needed?

- What features do I need the device or system to include?

- If other people are assisting me in the selection process, are they good at listening and do they seem open to new ideas?

- How will I consider and evaluate a range of possible solutions?

Gay wanted to increase her ability to write independently, instead of dictating to an attendant. She had been asked to contribute some movie reviews to an online journal. Her cerebral palsy made using a standard keyboard nearly impossible. By visiting a local assistive-technology lab, Gay found that with a programmable membrane keyboard, such as IntelliKeys, she was able to select individual letters, although slowly. Gay needed another piece of assistive technology in order to increase her entry speed. One of the options she tried was word prediction software. Based on the first letter or two entered, the screen would present a list of choices. For instance:

When Gay typed   *Ch_*

the software suggested

1. *Change*   2. *Charge*   3. *Challenge*   4. *Champion*

While this is a great option for some, it was not the best for Gay, as it required her to look and focus on the screen while typing. Given her physical abilities, it was faster if she could keep her focus mainly on the keyboard. Two other options would allow this. The first was an abbreviation expansion or "auto-correct" utility. This would allow Gay to enter frequently used words, such as *cinema*, along with a shortcut, such as *ci*. The software automatically changes the entry to the longer word. This would allow her to enter her entire name with two keystrokes. The only disadvantage to this method is that you need to remember the shortcuts. Since Gay would not be typing every day, there was a good chance she would forget the abbreviations. Gay's best option utilized the programmable nature of IntelliKeys. With assistance, she designed a keyboard overlay that put alphabet keys towards the lower right of the keyboard. In the space on the left and above, she added keys for entire words, such as her name, common terms used in movie reviews, and even word endings, such as *-ing*. This was the best solution, given her physical abilities and how often she would be writing.

Joey's teacher was concerned because his handwriting was slow, laborious, and difficult to read. His father was sure that a laptop would be the best solution, since Joey had been learning to type. His mother agreed but had concerns that a laptop was a big responsibility for a child entering third grade and that the laptop could get damaged or stolen. They asked the school about getting a laptop, and the IEP (individualized education program) team agreed to consider assistive-technology tools that would

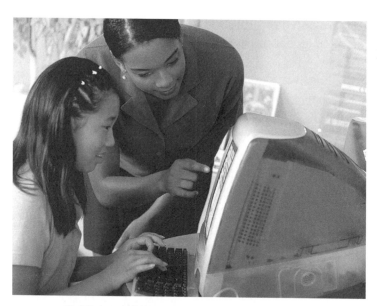

*Co:Writer 4000, a word prediction program and
Write:OutLoud, a talking word processor help struggling
students through the writing process
(Photo courtesy of Don Johnston, Inc.)*

assist Joey in producing the quantity of writing needed for third grade. The AT specialist for the school district was sent a package of information before meeting with Joey and his parents. She requested that Joey write a paragraph about his favorite sport. This took him seven minutes and produced three sentences with a total of eighteen words. Then she showed Joey a portable word processor. She asked him to write again, on another topic that he enjoyed. This time Joey produced five sentences in seven minutes, with a total of thirty words. The final trial was using a laptop computer that included a touch pad for moving the mouse, a word processor, and other programs. In this trial, he produced fewer sentences than with the portable word processor. This was due, in part, to the time it took to boot up the computer and to open the word processor.

The IEP team decided that the advantages of the portable word processor outweighed some of the additional features in the laptop. These advantages included the ability to start writing after pressing a single button, fewer distractions in the way of commands and other functions, a low profile on the desk that was consistent with the notebooks being used by other students, and the ability of the device to withstand bangs and blows.

Melinda is a different young lady today than she was three years ago. Then, she was a youngster with a lot to say but no way to express herself. She had learned in her short life that screaming in frustration was the quickest way to get attention. This method of communication had become her biggest barrier, and those working with her were as frustrated as she was.

During her first visit to an augmentative-communication clinic, it was suggested that she try a portable communication system consisting of a book of picture symbols. The occupational therapist and speech therapist suggested that the pictures in the book be color coded and provided ideas for how to use the book. Melinda's mother took these ideas and improved on them, attaching the book with suspenders, laminating it, and personalizing it for Melinda. At first, Melinda didn't use the book, and the challenge became one of how to facilitate her interest in this method of communication. One night Melinda was very upset and could not calm herself down. Her mom tried to help by asking Melinda what she wanted for breakfast the next morning. As she listed her daughter's favorite foods, Melinda became increasingly upset. She had a specific food in mind, but she couldn't communicate what it was. They went to the kitchen to try to find what Melinda desired, but she indicated it wasn't there. Then suddenly, Melinda remembered her communication book. She quickly retrieved it and pointed to a picture of a person eating a donut. They went out and got the donuts that night, and Melinda slept peacefully. So did her mom.

What resulted from these efforts was an enjoyable and functional method of communication. Melinda began actively communicating with her peers, friends, and family and showed much less frustration. Using signs, gestures, and verbal expressions along with her new book, Melinda became excited about communication and began making tremendous gains in school as well as at home.

A follow-up appointment with the augmentative-communication specialists was made because school personnel, Melinda's family, and the team believed it was time to add speech output to Melinda's total communication repertoire. After a school visit by the specialists, several different devices, all with voice output, were loaned to Melinda for trial periods of one to three months. She and her family determined the appropriate device. The one they chose, called EasyTalk, offered portability and lots of spaces for messages, and it was relatively easy to use. Mom reports that Melinda is enjoying her EasyTalk but that the learning process is never ending. Programming is ongoing because Melinda's communication needs are always changing, and Melinda sometimes cannot find what she needs on her board when she needs it. Still, the process itself has transitioned Melinda from a very unhappy girl to one who enjoys communication.

What do I need the technology to do?

Much of what individuals with disabilities want is simply access to conventional technologies or to accomplish daily tasks with greater ease or organization. You may want to be able to accomplish the following:

- Write with a word processor.

- Have teachers be able to read your writing.

- Explore the Internet.

- Publish a newsletter.

- Draw and experience the process of creating pictures.

- Create and perform music on a synthesizer.

- Play the latest computer games.

- Learn math with the help of a tutor.

- Send photographs to relatives and friends.

- Communicate with a range of people.

- Finish your homework.

- Make a movie.

- Remember appointments, assignments, or medication.

- Follow a recipe, even if you cannot read.

What are my strengths and weaknesses?

Assistive technology should capitalize on your strengths. For example, if you have difficulty reading but easily understand and remember spoken information, you might benefit from a system that changes printed words to computerized speech.

There are different ways to describe learning strengths or styles, including Howard Gardner's theory of multiple intelligences. Consciously or not, everybody draws on different styles at one time or another, but most of us find some modes easier than others. Learning styles and strategies include the following:

- **Auditory:** You remember what you hear and can follow oral directions.

  - You may benefit from hearing as well as seeing text, using a talking word processor, or using a text-reading program. You could tape-record lectures in order to later review the information.

- **Visual:** You understand information best when you see it; you can learn from reading.

  - You may benefit from written notes that convey a lecture. If you can't take notes yourself, the teacher can provide an outline or you can get a copy of another student's notes. You may benefit from seeing subtitles on a videotape.

- **Kinesthetic:** You learn by doing. You remember what you experience with your hands and/or body (movement and touch).

  - You may benefit from a simulation exercise, such as virtual frog dissection. Even moving around while you are listening can help increase retention.

Learning theories also talk about styles of processing information. These include the following:

- **Analytical:** You tend to see details of patterns more easily than the whole; you may prefer to learn step-by-step.

- **Global:** You tend to learn the general idea first, and then look at the details. You may prefer a less structured, more flexible environment.

Various resources are available to help you identify your learning strengths as well as to match your learning styles with different instructional technologies. To explore this area further, look for information on learning strategies, multiple intelligences, or learning style inventories at your local library or on the Internet.

What are the settings where the technology will be needed?

The right technology in one setting may be entirely wrong in another. You may need technology for work, school, home, the library, or even an afternoon in a café. Think about where you'll use it, whether it needs to be portable, how it will be set up or stored, and if you have the right furniture, cables, and lighting for it.

Home

The home can present some challenges related to the computer. Some people have little room in which to create a new work area. Adding a computer to the top of an existing desk will usually mean that the keyboard and mouse are too high and that the monitor is too low for an ergonomically correct setup. Raising the height of the chair is not recommended because your feet should be in contact with the ground, but it can be an option if you add an angled footrest. A keyboard tray may be a better solution, and a phone book can be used to raise the monitor. Removing the traditional desk and going with furniture designed for computers is often best. Check secondhand office-furniture outlets for bargains, where you may even find height-adjustable tables. These are great when multiple users are sharing a computer.

School

In a school, the primary purpose of assistive technology is to accomplish schoolwork—listening, note taking, reading, organizing, writing, test taking, and discussing. Some students also rely on assistive technology for communication. Here are some questions to think about if you plan to use assistive technology in a school setting:

- Will you need to share your equipment with others? If so, you may need an adjustable desk or chair; for instance, one that can also accommodate individuals who are still growing. Lighting in school environments can be harsh. Consider task lighting to help you focus attention or view a computer screen.

- Who is responsible for purchasing, maintaining, and/or replacing equipment?

- For very young users, consider a table close to the ground, where children can stand or sit on the floor or in small chairs. Consider where you'll locate printers, disk drives, and other components for ease of use. Computers and assistive devices can take up a fair amount of space on a tabletop or desk, and there should still be ample room for other materials such as books and papers. In many instances, especially with children, you'll need to insure that two or more people can work at the computer together.

Work

At work, the employer is under some obligation to offer employees an ergonomically correct work space. As in the home, this can be achieved by customizing the desk in order to get the keyboard and monitor at the proper height. (See the section titled "General Considerations and Ergonomics," below.)

Portable Systems

Will you do all your work in one location or do you need a portable system? A portable system may be more expensive and more prone to damage or theft, but it can offer greater convenience and flexibility, especially if you need a highly customized set of tools. Consider the following questions when contemplating purchase of a portable system:

- How will you transport it? You may need a case or, if you use a wheelchair, a sturdy mounting system.

- What parts will you need to take with you? What additional components might you need at home or work (a better monitor or keyboard, for instance, or extra cables and a power adapter)?

- Might it be cheaper and/or easier to have duplicate systems and to transport files by portable drive and/or e-mail?

- Do you need a full-fledged laptop computer or will a portable word processor or personal digital assistant provide the functions you need?

- Is the system you're considering compatible with existing printers, networks, and other devices in each setting (home, school, work, other)?

- Will you have the time (and help, if needed) to set it up or take it down in each setting? Extra batteries and wireless systems, such as Bluetooth, Airport, and WiFi, may be expensive but can eliminate the need to plug in and unplug cords or cables. Systems such as portable word processors and PDAs are less complicated to transport, set up, and use, and cheaper to replace if lost or broken.

- Does your existing insurance cover a portable system in each environment? You may need to obtain added protection against damage, loss, or theft.

- Will you need to use it outdoors? Be sure to check screen brightness, battery life, and water resistance.

- Will you be able to plug your system in or do you need long battery life?

General Considerations and Ergonomics

- Think about how to make your computer setup as convenient and comfortable as possible. Easy access and comfort are top priorities. The table surface on which you put the computer should be low enough so that when you sit you are looking down slightly at the monitor. If you are using a standard keyboard and mouse, your hands should rest comfortably on the desk and keyboard. Wrist rests and arm supports can help make your computing environment more healthful and comfortable.

- Will you place your monitor on top of or alongside the CPU? Or even on the floor, to provide access to young children? If more than one person or someone with a physical disability will be using the computer, consider a floating monitor arm. This is a mechanical arm that connects to a table and allows the monitor to move up, down, in, and out with ease, thus allowing people to change positions during the day and move the monitor into a position for best access.

- Positioning can be a complex issue for some people. You may choose to consult with an occupational or physical therapist who could help determine the best arrangement for you. If you need a customized setup—such as a way to mount a laptop computer on a wheelchair and use the chair's battery to run the computer—you might want to consult with an engineer or someone with the expertise to work with you. Many things can be fabricated to meet your needs. One resource for this type of expertise is the federally funded Rehabilitation Engineering Centers.

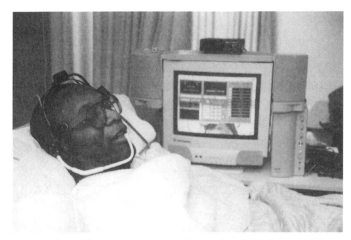

Assistive technology gives people greater control over their environment by translating actions such as head movement into computer commands. (Photo courtesy of Carolina Computer Access Center)

What features do I need the device or system to include?

It's time to start making a list of the specific features that you want to consider. Worksheet 4A, on the next page, offers some suggestions.

Check off the features that you believe you need. Then browse through the products in Part II, and use the column on the right to list product descriptions that seem like a good match. (The first group, software features, is simply a part of the standard computer operating system or software, such as the ability to change font, font size, and color in a word processor. The other four groups describe more specialized features.)

In terms of software features, do you need...	Product ideas from Part II, "Software Features"
☐ to get auditory feedback as you hit keys?	
☐ a way to reduce the sensitivity of the keyboard so that multiple letters do not appear?	
☐ icons as alternatives to word labels?	
☐ visual representation of auditory beeps or alerts?	
☐ an alternative to pointing and clicking?	
☐ a larger or more noticeable cursor or arrow?	
☐ the ability to customize many aspects of the content or interface?	
☐ Other:	

Worksheet 4A: Features I Need (cont'd.)

In terms of input to the computer, do you need...	Product ideas from Part II, "Product Descriptions: Alternate Input"
☐ a smaller or larger keyboard?	
☐ a keyboard with a different layout, fewer keys to reach for, or larger labels?	
☐ support to position the hand over a keyboard, mouse, or alternatives?	
☐ a way to type with only one hand?	
☐ a "virtual" keyboard on your computer screen?	
☐ a keyguard to prevent fingers from hitting the wrong keys?	
☐ a way to type by hitting a switch, moving the head, or other simple action?	
☐ a way to operate the system by voice?	
☐ a way to get paper-based images or text into the computer?	
☐ a hands-free operating mode?	
☐ to be able to simply touch the screen in order to select items?	
☐ an alternative to using a mouse?	
☐ Other:	
_____	
_____	
_____	
_____	

In terms of processing, do you need...	**Product ideas from Part II, "Product Descriptions: Processing Aids"**
☐ a way to use as few keystrokes as possible?	
☐ to increase the rate at which you can input information?	
☐ help in spelling?	
☐ help with skills development, such as math, writing, or reading?	
☐ text in outline format?	
☐ help with remembering things?	
☐ help locating, organizing, or retrieving information?	
☐ ways to "lock" part of the operating system or to get into a document more quickly?	
☐ Other:	
_____	
_____	
_____	
_____	
_____	
_____	
_____	
_____	
_____	
_____	

Worksheet 4A: Features I Need (cont'd.)

In terms of output, do you need...	Product ideas from Part II, "Product Descriptions: Alternate Output"
☐ large-print output?	
☐ spoken or auditory output?	
☐ Braille output?	
☐ enlarged text or images on-screen and/or in print?	
☐ more spacing between words, lines, and/or blocks of text?	
☐ the ability to see fewer lines of text at a time?	
☐ a more readable font?	
☐ enlarged images or a larger monitor?	
☐ electronic text or images in a portable format, such as on a PDA?	
☐ Other:	

_____

_____

_____

_____

_____

_____

_____

_____

In terms of more specialized systems and services, do you need a way to...	Product ideas from Part II, "Specialized Products"
☐ exchange typed messages (instead of voice messages) over the phone?	
☐ operate a variety of household electronics and lamps via a single control?	
☐ make hard-to-understand speech clearer when using the phone?	
☐ communicate without speech?	
☐ Other:	
_____	
_____	
_____	
_____	
_____	
_____	
_____	
_____	
_____	
_____	
_____	

If other people are assisting me in the selection process, are they good at listening and do they seem open to new ideas?

Let's consider who might have input into your selection process. Any user, young or old, may have strong preferences that influence the decision. Regardless of others' opinions, your own perspectives, ideas, and opinions about a particular solution or device are essential, or else it may never get used.

The perspectives of **family members, other caregivers, or, in some cases, friends and associates** may be needed if they will play a role in supporting the use of the technology. Some may be very eager to provide support, while others may want nothing to do with technology. Training for these supporters may be critical to the success of your chosen system.

Sometimes you may need to consult with a **medical professional**. For a communication device especially, a physician's prescription may be needed to obtain funding through Medicaid. Also, medical issues may impact selection. Is your condition stable? What changes can be expected, and what might be the rate and degree of change?

Many **schools** have designated a team of people to work on assistive technology. The team may include the speech and language pathologist, occupational therapist, physical therapist, teachers, or even an AT specialist. The parent(s) and the student should be welcomed members of this team.

For users with developmental or other disabilities, **social-services personnel or case managers** may be involved in coordinating benefits among agencies in order to fund assistive technology.

Some **manufacturer's representatives** were formerly assistive-technology specialists. They may be the best source of information on how elements of a system will work together, as well as on details for their particular product. As an added bonus, they often seek input and advice from users on how to improve future products.

Building rapport among team members is critical. It also requires tact. If there is disagreement within the team about a particular solution, propose a trial period and set a date and specific criteria for review. Both proponents and opponents of the selection know they'll have a chance to evaluate the decision before it becomes final. If you are working with professionals, vendors, or others, you may wish to monitor the following issues:

1. Are your perspectives and preferences as the user being considered?

2. Have alternatives been considered?

3. Are real data and the results of your hands-on trial being considered, as opposed to merely people's opinions?

4. Are your questions being answered respectfully and adequately?

5. Is the system under consideration as simple as possible while still addressing your goals?

6. Will the proposed system be sustainable over time in terms of training needs, setup, replacement parts, and other support?

How will I consider and evaluate a range of possible solutions?

There are two components to this question. First, let's consider ways in which you might gain access to specific technology devices.

Visit an **assistive-technology lab** that offers product demonstrations and trials. Labs can be found at Alliance for Technology Access centers as well as at some United Cerebral Palsy (UCP) facilities, disabled-student offices at universities or colleges, school-district facilities, independent-living centers, or state offices devoted to dealing with AT. Often such sites are dedicated to helping people select appropriate technology. You should find knowledgeable support and a wide range of products.

Visit a **public technology lab** that also offers AT, such as a community technology center or a public library. These may offer a more limited range of technology options, but they are still places to get hands-on experience.

Download **technology demo programs** from the Internet or order a demo CD from the manufacturer. Make use of offers such as 30-day free trials. This method requires you to visit each website or contact a number of manufacturers in order to compare products.

Work with **educational or medical professionals**, such as an occupational therapist, speech and language therapist, or others at your school, hospital, or other facility. Sometimes a team is available. Depending on their experience and access to AT products, this can be an outstanding way to try out a range of solutions.

Consult with an **AT products vendor**. Some vendors represent a wide range of solutions. Vendors for complex devices, such as augmentative communication systems, can offer an in-depth trial experience. A vendor may also be able to refer you to another customer who is successfully using a particular device.

Attend a **national or regional conference featuring AT**. Although sometimes hard to find, these events bring together a large number of AT vendors and AT users. Try an Internet search using the words "assistive technology calendar." Many AT conferences have special rates for consumers.

Consider **alternative strategies** or ways of learning about a particular product. For example, talk with **current users** in your community or in online communities, such as the ATA listserve, the QIAT listserve, or others (see Part III for a list of listserves and discussion groups).

The second component to this question is considering how you will evaluate options and features once you have tried them. Because it can be difficult to figure out what questions to ask, and it can be easy to forget what to ask, Worksheet 4B lists some questions to help you get started. The answers can assist you in narrowing your product choices. You might also want to compare features among various products. Worksheet 4C can assist with doing so. And finally, use Worksheet 4D as a checklist of questions to ask vendors when you're comparison shopping for AT.

Source: Adapted by permission from Dr. Marcia J. Scherer, Institute for Matching Person & Technology, Webster, New York.

Make enough photocopies of this worksheet so you have one for each different product you're considering.

Questions to Ask about a Specific Product

Each question below has two write-in spaces. Use the first one to indicate how important each question is for you or for this product. Use the second one to rank how well each question is addressed by the product. Use check marks, a 1–5 scale, or any rating system you prefer. Use a question mark to indicate where you need more information. Cross out any questions that are not relevant to your situation. Finally, use the space at the end to write down your own notes and questions.

PRODUCT NAME: _____

Importance   **Rating**

_____   _____ Does this product do everything I want it to do?

_____   _____ Does it require some skills or capabilities I don't have?

_____   _____ Once I learn the system, will I still need help from others to set it up or use it?

_____   _____ Will this technology meet my needs in various situations and environments?

_____   _____ Does the device have the features and stability I need in a variety of situations and environments?

_____   _____ Do I need to make changes in my environment(s) to accommodate my use of this device?

_____   _____ Will this product or system work with my existing equipment?

_____   _____ Can this product be adapted if there are changes in my functional abilities, activities, and/or size?

_____   _____ Are the controls, slots, etc., accessible and easy for me to identify and use?

Worksheet 4B: Matching Person and Technology (cont'd.)

PRODUCT NAME: _____

Importance   **Rating**

_____   _____ Are there extra features I should consider to make
the product more versatile?

_____   _____ Are there extra features that I'll never use?

_____   _____ Do I understand the maintenance schedule of the
device?

_____   _____ Is the average turnaround time for repairs accept-
able?

_____   _____ Is a loan available if doing without the product is
a problem?

Additional questions I want to keep in mind or address:

_____

_____

_____

_____

_____

_____

Important things to remember about using this technology:

_____

_____

_____

_____

_____

_____

_____

Worksheet 4C: Comparing Products

Use this worksheet to keep track of product features, sources, prices, warranties, and other key considerations. Make as many copies as needed to keep track of the products you're considering.

	Product 1	Product 2	Product 3
Feature(s) I need			
Training needs/ ease of use			
Compatibility/ system requirements			
Additional products or components needed to accomplish my goals			

Worksheet 4C: Comparing Products (cont'd.)

	Product 1	Product 2	Product 3
Price			
Vendor			
Contact person			
Phone/e-mail/web:			
Arrangements for hands-on testing:			
Other considerations			

Other qualities you may find important include:

Your age and gender, and the cultural appropriateness of the device.

_____

"Cool" factor: Do you feel comfortable with the way the technology looks, feels, and/or sounds?

_____

Speed of start-up and/or shutdown.

_____

Life span/obsolescence/upgrade options.

_____

Can the device meet current as well as anticipated needs?

_____

Vendor:

_____

Product:

_____

Contact person:

_____

Telephone, address, e-mail, website:

_____

On which computer system does your product operate?

_____

What version of the operating system does it require?

_____

How much memory (RAM) is needed?

_____

Are there specific monitor requirements?

_____

_____

Does the device need an external port on the computer to which it would connect by a cable? If so, what kind of port does it require?

_____

_____

Are all of the components I am considering compatible? Are there devices or brands of devices known to be incompatible with this device?

_____

_____

What are the key features of the product?

_____

_____

Worksheet 4D: AT Product Questions for Vendors (cont'd.)

How is this product different from other, similar products on the market?

_____

_____

_____

Do you have a distributor in my area, or do you handle your own
distribution?

_____

_____

How do the various types of these products differ?

_____

_____

_____

Do you feel you are qualified to work with me, knowing the features that I
find most important?

_____

_____

_____

What are my options for previewing this product to learn more about it?

_____

_____

Is it possible to obtain a short-term rental or loan of your product so that I
can explore it further and decide if it is right for me?

_____

If not, is there some other way I can try out the equipment?

_____

Other questions:

_____

_____

How Life Situations Impact Identifying and Selecting Technology

Unique considerations at each stage of life impact the process of planning for and selecting technology. Your current life situation may be addressed below.

Preschool

Early childhood settings typically offer a hands-on curriculum with a developmental rather than academic focus. These joyfully busy environments should easily accommodate children with differing abilities, but some school personnel may at first be unfamiliar or uncomfortable with using technology with children. Safety concerns are paramount. Be prepared to consider the following:

- Is the technology easy for children and their helpers to use?

- Is it developmentally appropriate (i.e., not too babyish for a four-year-old)?

- Does it support the child in engaging with others? Can other children also use the technology so the child learns alongside peers?

- Is it durable, spill resistant, and safe?

- Does it need to be moveable, storable, or lockable?

- Is there a "low-tech" alternative to consider?

Makenzie is a four-year-old with cerebral palsy. A few teachers and other parents were nervous about including him in a typical preschool. His mother and speech therapist worked with the head teacher to plan an afternoon for all the children and their parents to learn about the special strategies and equipment Makenzie uses to communicate and play. The children used a switch to make popcorn and a simple communication device to sing a song and to play red light/green light. Later, both parents and children were given a chance to ask questions and talk with Makenzie's family. These activities paved the way for Makenzie's full participation in the school.

K–12 (Public or Private)

Public laws such as IDEA (see Chapter 5) insure that students in grades K–12 will have access to a free and appropriate public education, including necessary accommodations to individualize their education as needed. Knowing your rights and building a good relationship with team members

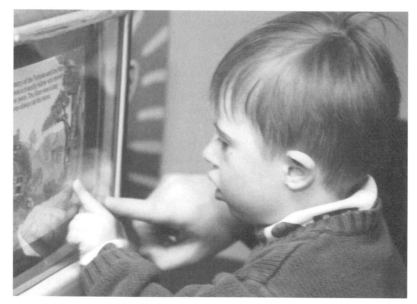

*This boy is reading a story using a touch screen on a computer monitor
instead of a mouse. (Photo by June Chaplin, courtesy of LINC)*

will contribute to the successful selection of appropriate strategies and technology. Be prepared to consider the following:

- Has the student been included in the process of selecting and reviewing the technology he or she will be using?

- Is the technology age-appropriate?

- Can the technology be used in ways that increase the student's inclusion and participation with peers?

- Does the technology increase the student's independence? Will the technology accommodate changes in the student's abilities and schoolwork demands?

- If needed for homework or communication, is the technology useful at home as well as at school?

- Will the student need access to the equipment year-round or just during school sessions? Is there a procedure for checking out school-owned equipment during vacation time?

- Will the student need a safe place to store and/or transport equipment?

- Who will purchase, support, maintain, and repair equipment?

- Is there a backup plan if the equipment breaks down or is left at home, lost, or stolen?

Maria was in fourth grade and still unable to write legibly or quickly enough to keep up in school. At home, she practiced keyboarding and did all her work on a computer, but at school, working on a computer often left her at the side of the room, with her back to class. Her family obtained a portable word processor on loan, and her teacher was so impressed with the possibilities for all her students that she convinced the parent-teacher committee to buy a set for general use.

Higher Education

Higher education often comes with new demands for independence, responsibility, and even technological literacy, yet many AT devices may be unfamiliar in academic settings. After years in the public school system, students may find themselves far from home and from familiar levels of support. Be sure to consider the following:

- If the technology is complex, are there timely sources of support?

- Are you prepared to explain, quickly and concisely, the need for the technology (e.g., during class lectures or exams), in the face of potential teacher resistance?

- Will the technology work with campuswide networks, labs, e-mail, Internet, or other information services?

- Many colleges or departments require students to own and use computers, often with a particular operating system or software. Does your system meet any such requirements?

Jeremy's political-science professor resented the fact that he came into class with headphones plugged into his laptop. Assuming Jeremy was setting up a new play list for his MP3 player, she lowered his participation grade and gave him a stern lecture. Jeremy appealed his low mark and showed her the text-to-speech note-taking software he was using. The next semester he demonstrated the system to his new professors before the term began.

In the Workplace

According to a study by the National Center for Disability Services:

> ...low-cost and low-tech devices often made the difference between having and not having a job. These might be items that most of us don't even

consider to be assistive technology. In fact they may be commonly used tools or pieces of office equipment like speakerphones that allow someone without hand use to access the telephone, or e-mail access that enhances communication for those who can't speak. In terms of personal characteristics, individuals cited their persistence and determination as important.

Back to Work (Reentry)

In the vocational rehabilitation (VR) process, one of the technology-related goals is to identify and resolve any problems that might prevent the VR agency from acquiring the technology you need. Working closely with your VR agent can greatly impact the success of your selection decision. For example, one particular model of a device may be approved for state purchase, but the version you need may not be.

At Home/Daily Living

You may want to contact your insurance agent to determine whether your homeowner's or renter's policy will cover your technology. If your general insurance does not cover computer equipment, check the phone book for companies that specialize in insuring personal-computer equipment. Also, if you are purchasing a laptop or portable computer, make sure your insurance carrier will cover it in all situations. We encourage you to consider this protection.

In the Community

Workspace and ergonomics are especially important when the goal is accommodating a wide range of needs. Mainstream technology has been moving increasingly in the direction of universal design. This means that mainstream hardware and software is useable straight "out of the box" or is customizable for use by a wide range of users with varying abilities and goals. Many organizations and agencies are also providing accommodations by adding commonly used assistive-technology products to their workstations. Ask any agencies that you work with about their access tools so that they are aware of your needs. Sometimes the assistive technology is available but not readily visible.

Injury, Illness

Assistive technology can be as important for individuals with temporary disabilities as it is for those with lifelong challenges. If this describes your situation, due to the shortened period that you will be using AT, consider choosing tools and strategies with quick learning curves, looking into loaner or demonstration options, and finding creative uses of existing or mainstream tools. For example, a talking photo album could function as a commu-

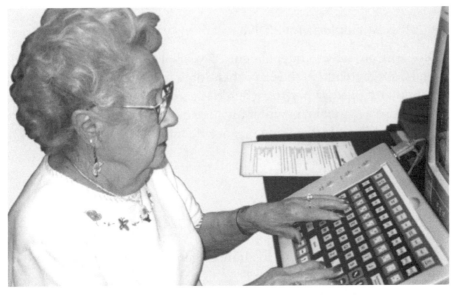

The world is becoming more accessible since products that were originally designed for people with disabilities are increasingly being used by others as well. (Photo courtesy of IntelliTools)

nication device for someone who's temporarily unable to speak. In addition, always consider the built-in assistive and productivity features of mainstream software before purchasing specialized tools.

Aging

According to a 1995 article by L. Gitlin in *Generations: Journal of the American Society on Aging,* "Assistive technology may be viewed positively, as a mechanism by which to regain independent performance, or negatively, as a symbol of lost function and abilities." Acceptance of assistive technology can be a difficult task if it's correlated with acceptance of a disability or if it's perceived as a negative social stigma. "I'm not blind, I just can't see" may be the attitude that the person wishes to maintain. Similarly, it's often difficult for an older individual to accept newer technologies, so a search for familiar motifs can help. Consider the following questions:

- Does the technology enable you to continue activities that have otherwise become difficult?

- Do you have a family member or friend who can help you with training or with technical troubleshooting?

- Are you willing to put time into learning a new way of doing things, such as writing with a computer?

- Is there a simpler solution that still meets your needs?

Olga was an active, independent 85-year-old when she had a stroke, which left her without the use of her dominant side. She learned to use a computer mouse by playing a familiar game of solitaire, yet she continued to use a manual typewriter for all of her letter writing and found her own way to knit by wedging one needle into the tightened crook of her right arm.

Worksheet 4E: Summing Up My Technology Needs

Now that you've considered the details involved in each of the steps outlined earlier in the chapter, you might use this worksheet to organize your thoughts.

What do I need the technology to do?

_____

_____

_____

What are my strengths and weaknesses?

_____

_____

_____

What are the settings or environments where it will be needed?

_____

_____

_____

What features do I need the device or system to include?

_____

_____

_____

If other people are assisting me in the selection process, are they good at listening and do they seem open to new ideas?

_____

_____

How will I consider and evaluate a range of possible solutions?

_____

_____

Chapter 5

The Law

What Are My Rights?

Robin Stacy, director of programs and services, Enabling Technologies of Kentuckiana, Louisville, Kentucky

The Big Picture

The U.S. Congress has passed several important laws that have the potential, when enforced, to greatly improve the civil rights of people with disabilities. Among many other benefits, these laws provide access to assistive and conventional technologies in certain situations for individuals with disabilities. Knowing your rights under the law will help you overcome any roadblocks you encounter during your planning for assistive technology.

Many people have taken this journey before you and have forged the way. The most significant trails blazed have been through the U.S. Congress. What follows is a review of the pertinent legislation enacted through the hard work and persistence of people with disabilities and their families, people who understand the growing importance of technology. The passage of these groundbreaking laws indicates that technology is gaining recognition at every level of our society and that advocates for its use are developing clout in every arena.

The goal of this chapter is to help you answer the following questions:

- What do all those acronyms stand for?

- Which laws pertain to me and how can they help?

- Whom do I contact when I have a problem?

Worksheet 5A, located at the end of the chapter, provides space for you to write down the answers to some of these questions as they apply to you. Having this information recorded in one place will serve as an important resource in your plan to gain access to appropriate technology.

Mike and Michelle are parents of three-year-old *Tommy*, who has autism. They were becoming more and more frustrated by Tommy's inability to use his voice to speak. At school and at home Tommy communicated by screaming, banging his head on the floor, or throwing things.

In desperation, Michelle asked other parents for suggestions and resources, and she was referred to a parent-training seminar. At the seminar Michelle heard about Tommy's legal rights and about something called "augmentative communication." She was also referred to her local assistive-technology center, where she learned more about augmentative communication devices and was able to borrow a device to try out at home with Tommy.

At home Michelle videotaped Tommy using the device. To demonstrate its effectiveness, she shared the video with school staff at Tommy's Individualized Education Program (IEP) meeting. Although the school staff at first resisted purchasing the device, Michelle knew about Tommy's rights to participate in the same activities as his peers. Armed with that information and with the video documenting Tommy's success using the device, she and Mike were able to persuade the school to give Tommy a chance to use a communication device in the same way that other children use their voices.

A Review of the Legislation

The laws described in this chapter include the following:

- Individuals with Disabilities Education Act of 1990 and 1998 (P.L. 101-476 and P.L. 105-17)

- Americans with Disabilities Act (P.L. 101-336)

- Assistive Technology Act of 1998 (P.L. 105-394) and the Technology-Related Assistance for Individuals with Disabilities Act of 1988 (P.L. 100-407), which was also amended in 1994 (P.L. 103-218) and is commonly referred to as the "Tech Act."

- Rehabilitation Act of 1973, as amended in 1992 and 1998 (P.L. 102-569 and P.L. 105-166)

- Telecommunications Act of 1996, Section 255 (P.L. 104-104)

By contacting the office of your U.S. congressional representative or senator, you can obtain copies of these laws and related background materials. Materials on all of these laws are available in Braille, large print, audiotape, and as computer files from the government agencies responsible for implementing and enforcing the laws, such as the U.S. Department of Education, the Justice Department, or the Federal Communications Commission. If you have access to the Internet, legislation can be located and reviewed through the websites operated by the Library of Congress and congressional representatives.

Keep in mind that you may not need all of the information given here for each law to help you determine a solution to your problem. In addition, be aware that laws may be amended, reversed, or otherwise altered over time, so it is important to stay current on legislation of importance to you.

As you read about the laws that pertain to you and your search for technology, think about the important role that advocacy can play in achieving your goals. Take note of the following points about advocacy:

- The laws form a good foundation for including technology as a regular part of your life, but none of them guarantee your access to technology.

- It is vital to learn about how the law applies to your particular life situation.

- Laws are only as good as we make them. Without enforcement, they become meaningless.

- If laws are violated and complaints are not filed with the authorities responsible for enforcement, violations will continue.

Advocacy can take the form of legal action, spoken or written formal complaints, or informal assistance that is intended to educate businesses or individuals who may not be fully aware of laws that prohibit discrimination on the basis of disability. Remember that in the fable about the wind and the sun arguing over which could best remove a man's coat, the sun (in the form of gentle action) won over the wind. Sharon's story illustrates this principle in action.

> *Sharon*, who uses a wheelchair, stayed at a national chain hotel and requested an accessible room. The room she was given was not fully accessible; a dresser blocked access to part of it. A call to the front desk brought employees to the room to rearrange the furniture so that she, or anyone else using a wheelchair, could move comfortably around the room.
>
> The hotel management was appreciative and asked Sharon to suggest other ways to make the hotel more accessible for people with disabilities. If the hotel had refused to make reasonable accommodations, Sharon would have taken more formal, legal action. Their willingness to cooperate and learn turned a tense and potentially litigious situation into one that had a satisfactory resolution for all.

Individuals with Disabilities Education Act (IDEA)

Originally titled the Education for All Handicapped Children Act of 1975 (PL-94-142), this law guarantees several basic rights and protective assurances for infants, toddlers, children, youth, and young adults with disabilities. These rights include the following:

- All children with disabilities are entitled to a free and appropriate public education (FAPE).

- To the maximum extent possible, children with disabilities should be educated with students without disabilities, as close to home as possible, and in the least restrictive environment.

- Children with disabilities must be provided supplementary services that permit them to benefit from their education, such as physical therapy and assistive-technology services.

- With the parents' informed consent, a fair assessment must be completed to determine the student's educational needs.

Early Intervention

In addition to provisions for the school-age population, the law includes requirements for infants and toddlers from birth to age three, as well as for young children ages three to five.

For infants and toddlers, assistive technologies may be specified in the Individualized Family Service Plan (IFSP). These may include adapted toys and other devices that develop readiness for computer-based technologies that the child will need in order to participate in the environment and to learn.

School Age

At age three, children are considered school aged and are mandated to receive services through their local public school system. In addition to the guarantees listed above, the following rights apply:

- Due process rights require that prior notice be given to parents before changes are made in the child's program and that a method be provided for resolving disagreements.

- Students who have been identified or who are perceived as having difficulty learning in school must have an IEP prepared annually for them by a team that includes the child's parents. The IEP must clearly spell out what services a student will receive and how and where the student will receive them, including specific educational goals and the tools to be used to accomplish these goals. An example of a specific goal would be, "John will write a well-organized, grammatically correct paragraph, free of spelling errors, using word processing software on a Macintosh computer equipped with IntelliKeys and a large-print overlay."

- Assistive technologies and technology access to the curriculum being used in the classroom *must* be addressed in the IEP. If a request for assistive technology is denied, the rationale must be presented in writing and is subject to appeal.

- Once assistive technology has been included in a student's IEP, the school system must provide it, as is true of any services included in an IEP.

- The Office of Special Education Programs of the U.S. Department of Education has issued a series of administrative letters over the years interpreting IDEA. One such letter stated that a school district or other local education agency may not maintain a flat policy barring the inclusion of assistive technology in IEPs. Rather, it must make a determination based on the facts of each case. Other letters have upheld the student's right to use assistive technologies purchased with school funds at home and away from school, when the IEP specifies that the devices are needed to maintain educational goals and learning.

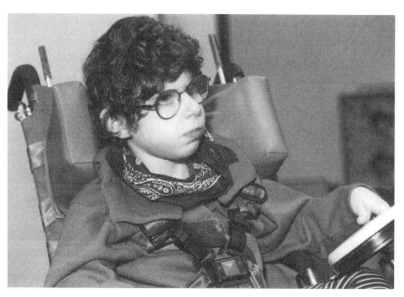

Simple assistive technology empowers individuals with disabilities. Here a student works with an Ablenet switch that allows for meaningful communication and participaton. (Photo by June Chaplin, courtesy of LINC)

Transition

IDEA mandates the inclusion of transition services in the IEP, beginning at age 14 and no later than age 16. Assistive technology can serve a vital role for youth with disabilities who are making the transition from secondary school to higher education, the workplace, or greater community involvement.

Note: IDEA is currently undergoing reauthorization. Some items described in this portion of the chapter may change as this reauthorization becomes law.

Americans with Disabilities Act (ADA)

Modeled after Section 504 of the Rehabilitation Act of 1973 and the Civil Rights Act of 1964, the ADA provides civil-rights protection against discrimination for individuals with disabilities. The protections afforded under ADA are similar to those provided in other legislation on the basis of race, gender, age, nationality, and religion.

- The ADA is described as the greatest legal landmark in the history of civil rights and equality of opportunities for America's estimated 54 million people with disabilities. Its impact upon the availability of assistive technology will be substantial.

- The ADA requires employers, governmental and nonprofit service providers, and businesses providing public accommodations to take reasonable steps to accommodate persons with disabilities.

- In the provision of "reasonable accommodations" or of the "auxiliary aids and services" sometimes required in public settings, equipment is clearly included among the strategies for meeting the law's requirements.

- While no business or organization can be made to provide accommodations that would create an undue financial burden or hardship, in many cases assistive technology represents the most appropriate and cost-effective method for meeting the need.

The ADA defines a *disability* as any condition that impairs major life activities, such as seeing, hearing, walking, or working. It covers nearly 900 specific disabilities. Under separate sections, it mandates accessibility and accommodation requirements in public facilities, in employment areas, at state and local government service facilities, on transportation services, and for communication purposes.

One of the protections afforded by the ADA that is not commonly discussed covers parents and guardians with disabilities who wish to participate in their child's school environment. PTA meetings, parent-teacher conferences, and other school events are required by law to be accessible. The law intends to break down the barriers that exist in all of these areas and to provide equal opportunity for individuals with disabilities.

- Among the many important rights and protections addressed in the ADA is the requirement that an employer with 15 or more employees may not discriminate against an individual with a disability when the person is qualified to perform the essential functions of the job, with or without a reasonable accommodation.

- The ADA defines *reasonable accommodation* as some modification in a job's task or structure, or in the workplace, that will enable the qualified employee with a disability to do the job.

- The modifications or changes, which can include the use of assistive technology and technology access, must be made, unless the change creates an undue hardship for the employer.

- Many employers and consumers (before doing their research) make the assumption that most modifications are going to be very costly and therefore qualify as undue hardships. This is not proving to be the case.

- Preliminary findings of the President's Committee on Employment of People with Disabilities indicate that the majority of accommodations cost less than $500, and many have little or no cost at all. This committee, a small federal agency, is working with businesses and groups representing people with disabilities to promote the successful implementation of the ADA.

- Where an accommodation or auxiliary aid or service is needed to meet the requirements of the law and no other defense applies, such as the cost constituting an undue hardship, the organization or business must provide it.

- This means that the business is obligated to pay for the technology, although the technology user may not become the owner of the equipment.

- One example of such an accommodation is the assistive listening devices used at public meetings.

The Assistive Technology Act and the Technology-Related Assistance for Individuals with Disabilities Act (Tech Act)

The Assistive Technology Act of 1998 is the amended version of the earlier Tech Act. It provides federal funds to assist states in developing easily available, consumer-responsive access to assistive technology, technology services, and information.

When signed into law in August 1988, the Tech Act was the first piece of U.S. legislation ever to use the term *consumer-responsive*. It requires that states must have a process for responding to the concerns and suggestions of citizens with disabilities.

The Tech Act provides a definition of *assistive technology* that has become the standard definition used in all subsequent federal legislation and regulations. *Assistive technology* is defined as "any tool or item that increases, maintains, or improves functional capabilities of individuals with disabilities."

- Assistive-technology categories include: daily living aids, positioning and seating, mobility, communication, computer access, and environmental control.

- In addition to "high-tech" devices, the Tech Act includes "low-tech" and "no-tech" devices, such as mechanical page-turners, custom-molded seats, single-switch-activated toys, and handheld magnifiers.

All states are funded to implement the Tech Act. States have primarily used their federal funds for providing technology services, such as information and referral programs and for creating statewide programs that provide access to assistive technology to individuals with disabilities.

In each state, the Tech Act agency can tell you about resources for funding the purchase of equipment. You can obtain information related to the Tech Act from the lead agency in your state.

The Tech Act is currently being considered for reauthorization. You can contact your state Tech Act agency for more information.

Rehabilitation Act Amendments of 1992 and 1998

In 1973, the Rehabilitation Act was passed. It was enacted to prevent discrimination against people with disabilities and covered employment and government services.

- The 1973 act primarily constituted a reauthorization of existing federal aid programs for people with disabilities. It provided a statutory basis for developing and implementing vocational rehabilitation and independent-living programs through research, training, services, and the guarantee of equal opportunities.

- In general, the Rehabilitation Act and subsequent amendments cover both public and private employment. The basic goals of sections 501, 503, 504, and 508 are to prohibit discrimination against individuals with disabilities and to increase their employment opportunities within society.

- The Rehabilitation Act amendments represent a dramatic departure from the practices that evolved in the rehabilitation system under earlier laws. Particularly for individuals with severe disabilities, the 1992 amendments abolish many barriers to gaining access to rehabilitation services.

- The former system evaluated individuals for their "employability," "feasibility of employment," and "rehabilitation potential." It served in many ways as the gatekeeper of opportunity for hundreds of thousands of people with disabilities.

- The 1992 law is built on the presumption of ability to achieve employment and other rehabilitation goals, regardless of the severity of disability.

- Under the 1992 law, "individuals with even the most significant disabilities should be presumed capable of gainful employment and provided the needed supports to do so."

- Vocational rehabilitation agencies are now required to focus on solutions and the attainment of employment outcomes.

- In a 180-degree shift in perspective, vocational rehabilitation agencies must provide services unless the agency can "unequivocally demonstrate" that no possibility of employment exists for a particular individual, even after careful consideration is made of every option for training, assistive technology, reasonable accommodation, and other supports.

- All state vocational rehabilitation agencies are required to provide a broad range of technology services on a statewide basis, and the technology needs of every client of a vocational rehabilitation agency must be addressed in the Individualized Written Rehabilitation Program (IWRP).

- Conceptually similar to the IEP required in educational settings, the IWRP for every client must contain "a statement of the specific rehabilitation technology services to be provided to assist in the implementation of intermediate rehabilitation objectives and long-term rehabilitation goals" (Minnesota Star Program, ADA/ADR Pilot Program 1996).

- On August 7, 1998, the president of the United States signed into law the Workforce Investment Act of 1998, which included the Rehabilitation Act Amendments of 1998. The amendments strengthened the law by requiring the federal government to make the technology it uses accessible to persons with disabilities as a part of Section 508 of the law. (Section 508 was originally added to the Rehabilitation Act in 1986; the 1998 amendments significantly expand and strengthen the technology-access requirements in Section 508.)

- Section 508 specifies that when federal departments or agencies develop, procure, maintain, or use electronic and information technology, they shall ensure that the electronic and information technology allows federal employees with disabilities to have access to and use of information and data that is comparable to the access to and use of information and data by federal employees who are not individuals with disabilities, unless an undue burden would be imposed on the department or agency.

- Section 508 also requires that "individuals with disabilities, who are members of the public seeking information or services from a federal department or agency, have access to and use of information and data that is comparable to that provided to the public who are not individuals with disabilities."

- The legislation exempts only national security systems from coverage of Section 508.

State Adoptions of Section 508 Guidelines on Information Technology Access

A growing number of states are passing legislation that adopts the Section 508 guidelines for state agencies. Maryland has said that Section 508 applies to all purchases made by school districts as well as to any websites they might produce. While these developments won't allow you to get your hands on personal assistive technology, they are being used as a means to ensure that more public technology and electronically based curricula are accessible, using features of universal design. This will increase compatibility with AT and in some cases even reduce the need for personal assistive technology. The Tech Act agency in your state should be able to tell you if Section 508 has been adopted in a way that would have an impact on educational technology.

Telecommunications Act of 1996, Section 255

Very much related to the goals of Section 508 of the Rehabilitation Act, the Telecommunications Act of 1996 requires all telecommunications systems and services to be accessible to members of the public with disabilities and also to federal employees with disabilities.

In a rapidly changing telecommunications environment, Section 255 contains specific language about how the telecommunications industry must

100

———

Computer
Resources
for People
with
Disabilities

change to enable people with disabilities to enjoy more of the benefits of new telecommunications technologies.

Section 255 mandates that all telecommunications products and services be "accessible to and useable by individuals with disabilities, if readily achievable." If not readily achievable, the products are required to be compatible with the assistive technologies and other adaptive equipment used by people with disabilities.

What to Do If You Have a Complaint or Problem

If you have a complaint about or a problem with accessibility or accommodation that you believe might constitute a violation of your rights, start by obtaining copies of the laws and related supporting materials, which are available from your congressional representative. In addition, other resources are available at the national and community levels.

Nationally

- There are ten federally funded resource centers called Disability and Business Technical Assistance Centers (DBTACs) that specialize in providing ADA information, training, and technical assistance to employers, people with disabilities, and other entities.

- Each state has a federally funded Protection and Advocacy (P&A) agency that receives funds under the Tech Act in order to include AT rights in their services. Your state P&A may have developed state-specific information about your rights in this area. P&A agencies have the authority to provide legal representation and other advocacy services, under all federal and state laws, to all people with disabilities (based on a system of priorities for services).

- Through the Attorney General's Office and the Office of Civil Rights, the U.S. Department of Justice places a high priority on fair, swift, and effective enforcement of the Americans with Disabilities Act. These agencies can help you receive lists of publications, location of the state or regional office nearest you, and information about people's rights and responsibilities under the law. They can also provide information about how and where to file a complaint.

In Your Community

Community-based advocates can help you figure out what steps to take next.

- Independent-living centers, parent-training and information centers, and consumer groups can be especially helpful.

- Parent centers can fully inform you about your options under IDEA and assist you in advocacy efforts.

- Independent-living centers and consumer groups can furnish you with a great deal of information related to ADA and the Rehabilitation Act amendments.

- Your state's department of vocational rehabilitation can provide materials related to the Rehabilitation Act amendments, and public schools are required to distribute information on IDEA to families who have children with disabilities.

Worksheet 5A: My Rights

Which laws pertain to me and how can they help?

_____

_____

_____

_____

_____

What are some of my personal concerns?

_____

_____

_____

_____

_____

What agency or organization will I contact?

_____

_____

_____

_____

_____

What questions do I want to ask?

_____

_____

_____

_____

_____

_____

Chapter 6

Funding Strategies

How Will I Pay for It All?

Janet Peters, ATA center director, PACER Simon Technology Center, Minneapolis, Minnesota

The Big Picture: Where You Are in Your AT Planning Process

In this chapter we focus on figuring out how to pay for the technology you need. Whether you are entering the process at this stage or have read earlier chapters in the book, consider the following:

- **Know which technology you want.** Have you selected the technology most appropriate for you? Are there alternate systems that can accomplish the same goal? Be prepared to explain and provide data for choosing a particular assistive technology to potential funding sources. Sometimes the type of equipment you choose will dictate the funding source. (Refer to Chapter 4 for information on selecting appropriate technology.)

- **Know the laws and your rights.** Are you aware of the laws and how they relate to assistive technology? Many laws govern funding resources for assistive technology. (Refer to Chapter 5 for information on laws pertaining to assistive technology.)

- **Know your budget.** What is your budget? Have you shopped around for the best price? Your ability to pay for all or part of the assistive technology will affect your funding strategy. (Refer to Chapter 7 for information on budgeting and buying.)

- **Know your long-term needs.** How long is the equipment designed to last? Is your funding source responsible for upgrades or will you need to pay? Understanding the longevity of your assistive technology will affect your funding strategy. (Refer to Chapter 9 for information on how to keep your technology working for you.)

104

Computer
Resources
for People
with
Disabilities

Useful Preparation

- Assemble in one place the worksheets from other chapters that you've already completed.

- If you are planning to seek funding from an organization or agency, take note of its requirements and begin to gather any necessary documents, such as proof of income, verification of eligibility, other applicable reports, and the like.

- Identify people you know who could help with the complicated funding process. Keep them posted on your goals and progress.

Steps to Consider

As important as the funding sources are, the imagination, persistence, and energy you bring to your search are even more important. Even while you recognize that obtaining funding may be challenging and that there are no simple answers, you must believe you can find a way to fund your technology dreams.

The remainder of this chapter will guide you through the details of locating funding resources. Think about the following points before you move ahead:

- Although your research on funding may happen simultaeously with your process of selecting assistive technology, it is important to know and be able to articulate your needs before approaching funding sources.

- Think about your budget for assistive technology. Do you need funding assistance with all of it or can you afford to purchase some devices yourself? Are you comfortable with loans or do you need grant funding?

- Document the entire process carefully. Keep a list of your contacts and take notes about your progress. Your records will be very useful, especially if you are working with more than one potential funder or if you need to appeal a case.

Paula was eight years old when her family decided to try to put together a home computer system. They wanted to give Paula an opportunity to become proficient in computer use and, ultimately, to become her own advocate. Her parents knew it would be difficult to find financial resources for the system they needed, and they anticipated that the school district would be difficult to convince to purchase a system appropriate for Paula's use, so they explored several avenues.

Because Paula was blind, her parents approached the local Lions Club, knowing of the club's interest in visual impairments. They discussed their needs with the club and borrowed the computer equipment they hoped to purchase so they could demonstrate it to some key members of the club. The members were captivated by Paula and by her technology, so they worked with the family to help them purchase the equipment Paula needed initially. As a thank-you, Paula demonstrated her new computer system to a packed crowd at the next Lions Club meeting.

Learn the Basics about Funding Sources

Your goals for technology will determine the equipment you select and how you prioritize potential funding sources. Once you've established your goals (see Chapters 1 and 2) and are on your way to figuring out which products you want (see Chapter 4), you will find it useful to begin collecting information on all potential funding sources as early as possible.

People use a wide range of funding resources to meet their assistive-technology needs. Many children and adults receive at least partial funding of assistive technology through national government-funded programs, while others use strictly local, nongovernmental sources. Still others use a combination of sources or pay for some equipment from their own personal resources.

How can you sift through all the information about the many potential funding sources available to you? Reading this chapter will serve as a good start. The next section describes a variety of funding sources—both governmental and nongovernmental. Since qualifying for funding is usually highly dependent upon a person's life circumstances, the list of sources is organized into categories relating to typical life situations, such as education, reentry into the workplace, etc. Information about the sources described in this chapter is conveniently summarized in the table "Funding Sources at a Glance." Finally, Worksheet 6A, located at the end of the chapter, will help you organize your strategy for pursuing funding.

Assistive technology is often funded within larger programs, such as special education or medical insurance. Vocational rehabilitation, special education, and Medicaid are the three largest governmental programs through which many adults and children qualify for services. The services and funding provided by these programs are available to those who meet the program's specific eligibility requirements. However, saying that someone is *entitled* to services is not the same as saying what those services will be. Services vary based on decisions the state makes about implementing the

106

Computer
Resources
for People
with
Disabilities

program, the availability of funds, and individualized assessments of need and potential. For example, an individual might receive Medicaid but might not be entitled to a particular medical procedure unless the state provides it and it is deemed "medically necessary" for the individual.

In many instances, particularly when several components are involved, funding will not come entirely from one source or all at one time. Some sources may provide funds for certain components, such the computer itself, while others provide funds for peripherals such as printers, assistive devices, software, or training. For this reason, your funding plan should identify and prioritize potential resources so that you can approach them in the most appropriate order. Doing so is important because a number of sources consider themselves "payers of last resort," meaning they won't pay until all other sources have either agreed or refused to fund. It is therefore critical to document the results, even when your funding request is denied.

For reasons such as these, obtaining financial assistance can be a complex matter. When pursuing funding for assistive technology, be aware that persistence, assertiveness, and imagination are often rewarded in extraordinary ways. Remember, the vast growth over the past decade in the availability of, awareness about, and use of technology devices has occurred largely as the result of grassroots efforts by people like you—people who wanted the equipment and found ways to acquire it. Be your own advocate, and don't be discouraged by attitudinal or systemic barriers you may encounter in your search. Systemic barriers—those that relate to administrative and bureaucratic obstacles—are particularly difficult to overcome. Examples of systemic barriers might include agencies that provide access to technology, but only for specific types of applicants or only for specific or limited activities. The funding landscape is filled with systemic barriers. Working to remove them is an important effort for advocates and consumers of assistive technology.

Learn the Criteria

Generally speaking, funding sources can be organized according to their criteria, which may include any or all of the following:

- Your purpose for using the technology (such as vocational, educational, communication, quality of life, independent living, or medical necessity)

- The nature of the equipment

- Your age

- Location requirements

- Financial circumstances

The chances of persuading people or organizations to do what you want increase with your ability to meet their criteria, to follow their procedures, and to use their language. You should research potential funding sources thoroughly. Find out what they need to know.

Funding sources will have different and sometimes complex sets of selection criteria. Review the eligibility criteria carefully; don't dismiss a potential source until you are certain it will not work for you. For instance, many programs use "means testing," which is a way of determining eligibility for a program or service based upon income, resources, or other measures of individual or family economic status. Within the means test, however, some things may be exempt. Until you know exactly what goes into a particular agency's calculations for the means test, you should not assume you are ineligible.

The language you use with different funding sources should reflect the orientation of the source. Remember, it is important to research and understand the language the potential funding source prefers. Here are some examples of what we mean language concerns:

- In **medical** settings, stress the therapeutic nature and "medical necessity" of the equipment.

- In **vocational** settings, the goal of and potential for employment and self-sufficiency are crucial elements.

- In **educational** settings, the technology needs to help achieve academic and educational goals.

- In **urgent** or **time-sensitive** situations, service organizations that have more flexibility may offer the best options.

Sometimes vendors (companies who supply the goods and services you want) can help you understand what is needed to obtain authorization from an agency or insurance company.

Consider Cutting Costs

The cost of the technology is important to many potential funding sources. Opportunities to cut costs should be explored and may even generate increased interest from a potential funding source. You will want to evaluate product features in relation to cost.

Purchasing used equipment is one way to save on costs. Particularly in the computer field, fast-changing technology and continuous user upgrades can result in the availability of good-quality used equipment at attractive prices.

108

Computer
Resources
for People
with
Disabilities

However, it is important to keep in mind what you want to accomplish with the technology, or you may end up with a "bargain" that doesn't meet your needs.

How Life Situations Impact Funding

Qualifying for government aid for assistive technology is heavily dependent on your life situation. The first part of this section describes specific governmental programs based on various life situations. The second part of the section describes several nongovernmental sources.

Many governmental sources of funding have an appeals process. In fact, appealing funding decisions is quite common. Don't be deterred by an initial denial, as many appeals for funding of assistive technology are eventually successful.

Preschool and K–12 (Public)

Special Education

Special-education programs are administered under the Individuals with Disabilities Education Act (IDEA) and include a variety of services that school systems must provide so that students with disabilities receive a "free and appropriate public education."

IDEA has two parts:

1. Part C, Infants and Toddlers with Disabilities, covers children from birth to three years old.

2. Part B is for individuals from three to 22 years of age. Children with disabilities may be eligible for assistive-technology funding through special education in the public school environment.

The process to qualify for special education involves the following steps:

- The first step is a referral for screening and evaluation. Anyone can initiate the referral, but usually a parent, teacher, or related service provider (occupational or physical therapist, etc.) starts the process.

- A decision is then made about the need for special-education services.

- If a child qualifies, an Individualized Education Program (IEP) team convenes to determine the needs of the child, such as school placement, services, and equipment. The IEP team members include the child's parents, at least one teacher who may be a general or special-education teacher, at least one administrative staff person, and the child, when appropriate. The child's needs and the implementation plan are documented in the IEP and reviewed annually.

Every child with an IEP must be considered for assistive-technology devices and services. If the IEP team determines that assistive technology is needed for a "free and appropriate public education," it must be provided by the school district. The school may use nonschool funding sources, such as a supplemental grant. However, the school is ultimately responsible for providing the documented assistive technology, including services and aids, whether or not it finds additional funding.

Parents are IEP team members. Students are invited to participate during the transition process or sooner, and their opinions must be sought. Parents and students have important rights in the process, including the right of participation, the right to have experts of their own choosing at the IEP conference, the right to administrative appeal, and even the right to court appeal if they are dissatisfied with the administration's decision.

A 504 Plan

If a child does not meet special-education criteria, it is possible to acquire needed devices through a 504 plan. Section 504 of the Rehabilitation Act mandates that any program that receives federal funds, such as public schools, may not discriminate against any person on the basis of a disabling condition. Students with disabilities must be given the same opportunities to participate in educational programs and activities as students without disabilities, and the use of assistive technology may be considered as an accommodation. For example, a student with poor handwriting may use alternative methods, such as using a word processor or a computer.

Section 504 does not require school districts to develop an IEP for students. However, the district should document, in a written 504 plan, what evaluations were performed and what decisions were made regarding the student.

K–12 (Private)

Private schools that do not receive federal funds are not required to provide special-education services or other accommodations to children with disabilities, beyond the accessibility outlined in the Americans with Disabilities Act (ADA).

However, IDEA mandates that a student who would be receiving special-education services on an IEP if they were attending public school must be provided the same amount/proportion of special education and related services as would be federally funded to the public school. The formula is determined on a state-by-state basis. Ask for your state's funding formula from the department of education.

110

Computer
Resources
for People
with
Disabilities

Many private schools provide excellent services for children with disabilities, including funding for assistive technology. For information on services for children with special needs, contact the school administrative office.

Higher Education

The key to a successful postsecondary education is for students to become knowledgeable about their own accommodation needs and education responsibilities. Although protections against discrimination exist, college and university students have greater responsibility for initiating, designing, and ensuring their own accommodations.

Americans with Disabilities Act (ADA)

The Americans with Disabilities Act of 1990 (Title II) and Section 504 of the Rehabilitation Act of 1973 prohibit discrimination on the basis of disability. Practically every postsecondary school in the United States is subject to one or both of these laws, whose requirements are similar.

Unlike services provided in K–12 public schools, postsecondary institutions are not required to provide a "free and apppropriate public education." Rather, a postsecondary school is required to provide educational supports and reasonable accommodations as necessary to students with disabilities to ensure equal access to educational opportunities. Appropriate academic adjustments may include assistive technology.

The appropriate academic adjustment must be determined based on the disability and individual needs. Often such accomodations are not individually prescribed devices. For example, a postsecondary school could have specialized software, like a screen reader, available in a computer lab, but not purchase the technology for a student's private use. The computer lab equipment would qualify as an accomodation.

In the Workplace and the Community

ADA

The ADA requires employers, governmental and nonprofit service providers, and businesses providing public accommodations to take reasonable steps to accommodate persons with disabilities.

Where an accommodation is needed to meet the requirements of the law, the organization or business must provide it. Such an accommodation may be assistive technology. There are exemptions to providing an accommodation based on "undue hardship," a hardship potentially caused to the employer, agency, or business.

If a business is required to provide technology as an accommodation, the person with a disability does not become the owner of the equipment. One example of such an accommodation is the assistive-listening devices used at public meetings.

Workplace Reentry and Transition from School to Work

Vocational Rehabilitation

Operating through state agencies under the auspices of the Federal Rehabilitation Act of 1973 and Amendments of 1998, vocational rehabilitation programs (called by a variety of names, such as VR, DRS, OVR, or DR, depending on the state) provide assessment, training, job placement, and other services to people with physical or cognitive disabilities. To qualify for vocational rehabilitation, one must have a physical or mental condition that makes it difficult to prepare for, obtain, or keep work. Nationally, the VR programs have an "order of selection" whereby priority is given to individuals with the most functional limitations in the areas defined by the Rehabilitation Act.

For qualified individuals, services are planned and provided according to an annual contract between the agency and the recipient, called the Individualized Plan for Employment (IPE) or Employment Plan (EP), depending on the state.

Assistive technology can be written into the IPE in two ways. First, rehabilitation technology may be designated as one of the services that must be provided. Second, technology may be deemed to be part of another service, such as job placement.

Although the law requires an IPE, many adults in the rehabilitation system are unaware of the requirement. If you are using rehabilitation services, check to make sure you have a current IPE in place.

In the VR process, there are three technology-related goals:

1. To ensure that all eligibility determinations take full account of technology's potential to help achieve program goals;

2. To ensure that temporary technology (technology to be used until you obtain the proper long-term technology) is incorporated into the IPE in a timely way so that it is available when it is needed for employment or other life events;

3. To identify and resolve any problems that might prevent the VR agency from acquiring the technology you need. For example, one particular model of a device may be approved for state purchase, but the version you need may not be.

112

Computer
Resources
for People
with
Disabilities

Social Security

There are two programs under Social Security that offer work incentives that may help fund assistive technology. To qualify for Social Security Disability Insurance (SSDI), a person must have once worked but can no longer do so because of a permanent disability that affects the person's ability to work now or in the future. Disability is based on a doctor's diagnosis and the prognosis of ability to perform future work.

A person can receive Supplemental Security Income (SSI) at any age based on a doctor's diagnosis or disability. Using this method is complex, however, because added income could jeopardize benefits.

If you choose to fund your assistive technology through SSI or SSDI, it is vitally important to fully understand the work-incentive rules. These rules can be used to leverage work- and training-related technology for people who could lose their benefits if they obtain the equipment through personal resources.

The Social Security Administration offers publications that provide detailed descriptions of incentives and their potential impact on benefits and opportunities. The National Assistive Technology Advocacy Project publishes *Work Incentives for Persons with Disabilities under the Social Security and SSI Programs* (August 2002), a worthwhile resource.

The Social Security Administration's website (www.ssa.gov) also contains the most current information and changes related to work incentives. Finally, remember that knowledge is power and that you have the right to appeal any work-incentive plan that is denied.

At Home/Daily Living

Medicaid

Medicaid was established under Title 19 of the Social Security Act and is administered by state agencies. Medicaid is a national program of medical assistance for the poor, including people with disabilities. The program is income-based and covers people of any age, but only if the person or the person's family qualifies as low-income. Medicaid will purchase, rent, or lease various types of assistive devices called "durable medical equipment" (DME) for Medicaid beneficiaries if the devices are considered medically necessary. Generally, that means the equipment must be:

- prescribed by a physician
- used to restore or approximate normal function of a missing, malfunctioning, or malformed body part

- directly related to a diagnosed medical condition

- expected to provide a therapeutic benefit

Medicaid has appeals processes, both for ineligibility determinations and for decisions relating to the scope of services. Appeals can take time, but usually must be completed within 30 to 60 days. Guidelines regarding the appeals process and the required time frame can be obtained from your state's Medicaid office.

Medicare

Medicare is a federally funded health-insurance program for Americans over 65 and people under age 65 with severe disabilities of a certain duration. Medicare will help pay for health-care costs for individuals who qualify for the program. Medicare has two parts: Part A, Mandatory Hospital Insurance, and Part B, Optional Medical Insurance.

Part B can pay for durable medical equipment (DME), including assistive technology. Medicare will purchase various types of assistive devices if they are prescribed by a physician, supplied by a Medicare provider, and medically necessary.

Veterans Administration

The Veterans Administration funds communication devices that are prescribed for a person who has a disability related to military service. Other funding projects vary. For further assistance, call the Veterans Administration in your area.

The Tax System

A number of provisions in the tax laws can translate directly into financial assistance for individuals trying to acquire assistive technology. Favorable tax laws can lower the net cost of technology for individuals and families. In fact, by making sure you can justify the purchase, by keeping adequate documentation, and by paying attention to the timing of the expenditure (in relation to the tax year), you can deduct much of the cost of assistive technology—and virtually all of the cost of items designed or modified for use in the context of a disability—either as medical expenses, impairment-related work expenses, or architectural or transportation barrier–removal expenses. Consult with a tax specialist about your specific rights.

Nongovernmental Funding Sources

In addition to the governmental programs listed above, there are many local, private, and specialized nongovernmental sources that fund assistive technology.

114

—

Computer
Resources
for People
with
Disabilities

Community Service Organizations

In many communities, service, religious, or fraternal organizations, such as the Elks and Lions clubs, provide equipment directly to individuals under particular circumstances. Small, case-by-case grants of this sort are hard to categorize, but they tend to hinge on the applicant's ties to the community.

Foundations

Some private foundations address disability-related needs on an ongoing basis. Foundations, however, are far more likely to give grants or loans to organizations than to individuals. When they do fund individuals, the priorities are often higher education, medical care, or disaster relief.

Foundation directories can be found in public libraries or in the libraries of foundation offices.

Commercial Loans

Commercial credit is becoming more widely available for the purchase of assistive technology. Loans may be available through traditional lending institutions, consumer and membership groups, nonprofit organizations, or joint efforts between device vendors and banks.

At least fourteen states have received federal funding to establish financial loan programs for individuals with disabilities to purchase assistive technology. The states include Arizona, Arkansas, Florida, Illinois, Kentucky, Louisiana, Maryland, Michigan, Nevada, Oklahoma, Pennsylvania, Utah, Virginia, and Wisconsin. Many other states are independently supporting such programs.

Here are some questions to consider before applying for a loan:

How comfortable are you with debt? A loan is much different from a grant. Defaulting on debt can affect your future credit rating.

How much money do you need to borrow? The dollar limits for loans will vary, but a typical loan for assistive technology is $10,000 to $30,000.

What interest rate and repayment terms can you afford? Interest rates vary widely from low or no interest to a high rate. Some loans may offer interest rates below the federal prime lending rate to people with disabilities. The term for repayment typically ranges from five to seven years.

Is your credit history good? Problems in an applicant's credit history from interruption of earning power due to the onset of disability or from other, unintentional causes or actions that were not deliberate must be pointed out and explained to the lender.

Make your loan case as strong as possible. Lenders especially like to hear if the equipment is directly linked to improved employment. Put your best case forward.

Private Insurance

Private medical insurance comes in many forms and is still largely unregulated when it comes to assistive technology. Although insurance companies do purchase some assistive technology, insurance plans and policies are often silent about exactly what technology is covered. Technology and services must be medically necessary in order to be covered by these plans.

While a typical insurance policy will cover dependent children only through a certain age or until they complete college, many policies have special provisions to cover adult disabled children indefinitely. Check with your employer's benefits department regarding the company policy on covering dependents with disabilities.

Telecommunication Equipment Programs

Programs for access to telecommunications equipment provide devices needed by people with hearing, vocal-communication, motion, visual, or other disabilities so that they can use the telephone network. Available equipment includes speakerphones, text telephones (TTYs), phones with large buttons, and amplified phones.

Funded by fees of a few cents a month charged to all telephone users, these programs vary from state to state in terms of who and what they cover, both in their use of means tests and in other respects. To date, the programs have been largely limited to basic telephone access. Whether they will eventually extend to more advanced communications technology, only time and advocacy will tell.

The simplest way to learn if your state has such a program is to check a telephone bill. The programs are described differently from state to state. In California, for example, the program is called Communication Devices Funds for Deaf and Disabled. Contact your local phone company to inquire about its programs.

Finding More Funding Information

Don't go it alone! Many local and national nonprofit organizations offer information and expertise in navigating the bureaucratic maze of funding. These might include the following:

> **The Alliance for Technology Access (ATA)** provides information and referrals to individuals with disabilities, their family members, and others interested in assistive technology.

116

Computer
Resources
for People
with
Disabilities

United Cerebral Palsy Associations, Inc., (UCPA) provides funding information to individuals with disabilities, their family members, community-based organizations, and others.

Independent-living centers offer insight, guidance, advocacy, and technical assistance. They can be a vital link in the funding chain, particularly as a networking source.

Each state has a **Tech Act Project**, funded through the federal Assistive Technology Act. Services vary from state to state, but all include information-dissemination activities. Several programs have compiled statewide funding-resource directories. Federal funding for the Assistive Technology Act is scheduled to end in 2004.

Ten regional **Disability and Business Technical Assistance Centers (DBTACS)** serve the nation. They operate toll-free information lines for answering questions about the ADA and also provide information on assistive-technology funding.

Parent Training and Information Centers (PTIs) in each state provide training and information to parents of infants, toddlers, children, and youth with disabilities and to professionals who work with them. PTIs are specifically qualified to offer information about the Individuals with Disabilities Education Act (IDEA), including information on the funding of assistive technology.

Funding source	Age requirement	Scope	Life situation/other typical qualifying criteria
A 504 Plan	All ages	National	• Public school K–12
ADA	All ages	National	• In the workplace and community
Commercial loans	18+ (person applying)	Local	• At home/daily living • Determined by the user
Community service organizations (e.g., Lions Club)	Specific to organization	Local	• Time-sensitive • Not covered by other sources
Private foundations	Specific to organization	Local (but can vary)	• Higher education • Medical need • Disaster relief
Medicaid	All ages	National	• Medical need • Low-income
Medicare	65, or has had a disability for two+ years	National	• Medical need
Private insurance	All ages	Local/ regional	• Medical need
Social Security	All ages	National	• Workplace reentry • Transition from school to work
Special education	Part C: birth–3 Part B: 3–22	National	• Preschool • Public school K–12 • Transition from school to work
Tax incentives	18+ (person applying)	National/ state	• At home/daily living
Telecommunication Equipment Program	All ages	State	• At home/daily living
Veteran's Administration	18+ (veterans)	National	• At home/daily living • In the workplace and community
Vocational Rehabilitation	14+	National	• Workplace reentry • Transition from school to work

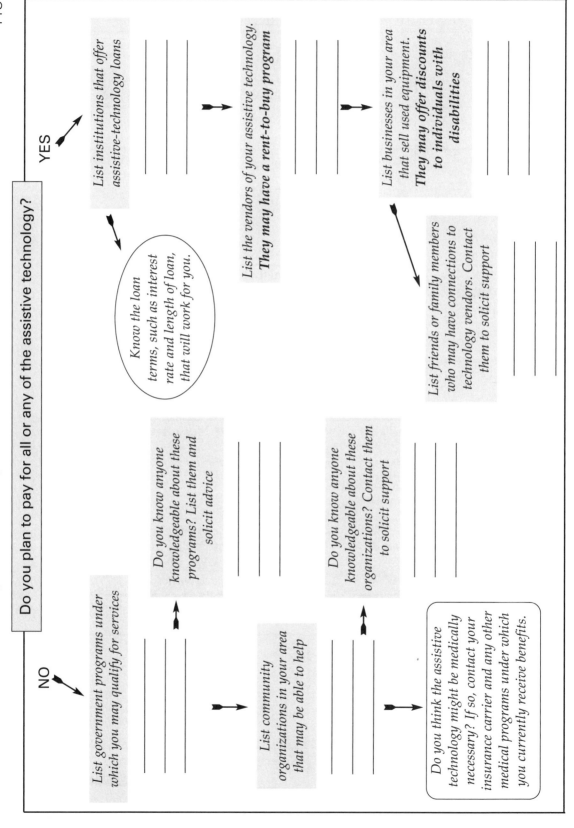

Worksheet 6A: Planning for Funding

Do you plan to pay for all or any of the assistive technology?

YES

List institutions that offer assistive-technology loans

_____
_____
_____

Know the loan terms, such as interest rate and length of loan, that will work for you.

List the vendors of your assistive technology. **They may have a rent-to-buy program**

_____
_____
_____

List businesses in your area that sell used equipment. **They may offer discounts to individuals with disabilities**

_____
_____
_____

List friends or family members who may have connections to technology vendors. Contact them to solicit support

_____
_____

NO

List government programs under which you may qualify for services

_____
_____
_____

Do you know anyone knowledgeable about these programs? List them and solicit advice

_____
_____
_____

List community organizations in your area that may be able to help

_____
_____
_____

Do you know anyone knowledgeable about these organizations? Contact them to solicit support

_____
_____
_____

Do you think the assistive technology might be medically necessary? If so, contact your insurance carrier and any other medical programs under which you currently receive benefits.

Budgeting and Buying

Where Should I Shop and How Much Will It Cost?

Jane Berliss-Vincent, director of adult/senior services, Center for Accessible Technology, Berkeley, California

The Big Picture: Where You Are in Your AT Planning Process

In this chapter we focus on selecting a vendor for you to work with and creating a budget for purchasing equipment. First, you might reflect on other aspects of your AT plan that could directly influence the way you approach this phase. Whether you are entering the process at this stage or have read though other chapters in this book, consider the following:

- **Know your funding strategies.** Have you developed a funding strategy to pay for the technology? Your funding strategy may impact the products you can afford to purchase. (Refer to Chapter 6 for information on funding strategies.)

- **Know what equipment you want to purchase.** Have you selected the type of equipment you want and had preliminary discussions with vendors? (Refer to Chapter 4 for information on selecting equipment.)

- **Know the laws and your rights.** Are you aware of the laws and how they relate to your options for obtaining equipment? (Refer to Chapter 5 for information about the laws and your rights.)

- **Assess your technology needs and set your goals.** Are you clear about what you want to be able to accomplish with the support of technology? This will impact which technology to purchase. (Refer to Chapter 2 for suggestions on how to assess your needs.)

- **Determine your training needs.** Have you identified any training you may need in order to be able to use your equipment (including computer basics, use of applications such as word processing or the

120

———

Computer
Resources
for People
with
Disabilities

Internet, and use of any assistive technology)? This will influence how well you are able to use your technology and may require additional funds. (Refer to Chapter 8 for information on how to determine your training needs and options.)

- **Determine your needs for technical support.** Have you identified what resources are available to you if your computer breaks down or your software doesn't work right and whether you will need to pay to use them? (Refer to Chapter 9 for information on how to plan for technical-support needs.)

Useful Preparation

We have provided worksheets in this chapter to help you organize your budgeting process. You may wish to make copies of them so you can keep track of your process and take notes.

Use the standard computer configuration as a starting point. In the final budget you may modify the configuration based on your needs and the requirements of the hardware and software that you will be using.

While price is a major consideration in selecting a vendor, it should not be the only consideration. Worksheet 7A includes a list of questions for you to ask vendors to help you determine their knowledge about their products, the support programs they offer following purchase, and your comfort level in talking to them.

You will likely have one of two budgeting styles: either listing all the equipment you want and finding funding for the total amount, or starting with a funding limit and listing equipment that will fit within that limit. Worksheets 7B and 7C address each of these styles. If you want to create a multiyear budget, make additional copies of the appropriate worksheets.

Be aware of the following resources, which may be helpful in guiding you through the development of your purchasing plan:

- Community-based assistive-technology sites are usually objective places to learn about people's experiences with particular vendors, brands of available technology, etc.

- Several online databases of product information exist to help you research product capabilities and prices.

- Most vendors have websites and/or catalogs that can help you make your decision.

Steps to Consider

The remainder of this chapter will guide you through the details of budgeting for and purchasing technology. As you read, bear in mind the following questions (some of which the chapter will help you answer for yourself):

- What pieces of technology (assistive and conventional) are essential to meeting my needs?

- Which are important, but not essential? Which are convenient, but not essential?

- Which vendor(s) that I've spoken with would I feel most comfortable buying from?

- What support services—computer setup, training, etc.—will I need?

- What ongoing expenses associated with my computer use—e.g., Internet account—will I have?

- What long-term budgeting needs—e.g., planning for equipment upgrades—do I want to consider at this time?

Lucille runs a home-based business; she handles pension plans for small businesses. Since she was diagnosed with macular degeneration in 1992, she has used a computer to store client records on spreadsheets. She also uses word processing software to create outlines for Bible-study classes at her church.

Recently, Lucille's 10-year-old Macintosh computer stopped working, and she needed to make decisions about acquiring a new computer. She was reluctant to change to a Windows operating system because doing so would mean learning a new platform and possibly new applications. However, her visual acuity had changed, and the available Macintosh options did not meet her magnification needs. After spending some time talking with her local ATA center and with other resources about her options, she decided to buy a Windows-based computer.

Because she was purchasing an entirely new system, Lucille took advantage of the opportunity to create a budget that included all the equipment that would be helpful to her. For example, because she had to buy a new printer, she decided that she wanted one that also had fax and scanning capabilities. This option proved not only more economical, but also made better use of Lucille's available office space. She had also gotten used to having a trackball rather than a standard mouse, and she wanted a Windows-compatible version of the model she liked. When she found out that the trackball was no longer commercially available, she

122

Computer
Resources
for People
with
Disabilities

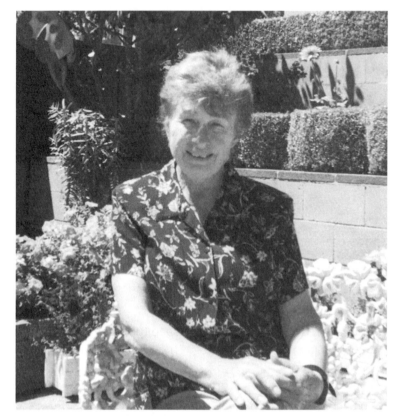

Lucille

got advice from vendors about similar models and included them in her final budget.

When Lucille was still considering acquiring another Macintosh computer, she found only one vendor who was able to provide both a new computer and the assistive technology she needed. Lucille had a positive experience working with this vendor, even though she ultimately decided to buy a Windows-based system. Consequently, even though there were other vendors who could have met her requirements, she decided to stick with the vendor who had already proved helpful.

Fortunately, Lucille did not need to budget for training or computer setup. She is lucky enough to have supportive family members living nearby who have computer expertise, so she did not have training expenses. The vendor she worked with brought her new equipment to her house and set it up at no additional charge, so she did not need to include a fee for the initial setup in her budget.

Find the Right Vendor for You

New assistive technology is usually sold through one of the following four channels:

1. Many types of assistive technology can be purchased directly from the manufacturer. This type of vendor is usually (but not always) the most knowledgeable resource about equipment features, system requirements, compatibility issues, upgrade schedules and policies, and other important information. Even if you decide to purchase the equipment from a different source, it is a good idea to contact the manufacturer and ask the manufacturer's support staff any critical questions.

2. Assistive-technology vendors often have authorized dealers in multiple locations. These dealers may be able to provide "value-added" services such as product-upgrade funding programs unavailable to nonauthorized dealers.

3. Independent dealers may lack access to the same benefits as authorized dealers. However, they are still worth considering, since they may be equally knowledgeable and supportive, and they may provide their own range of value-added services.

4. Sometimes there is only one source for purchasing a given product. Even in this case, you want to make sure that the dealer meets your quality standards. In some situations you may find it preferable to purchase a product with fewer features but better vendor support over a more complete product whose dealer makes you feel uncomfortable.

You may have the option of either buying both your computer and assistive technology from an assistive-technology vendor or buying the computer from one source and the AT from others. Use the budgeting worksheets to compare all the associated costs involved in these two approaches, not just the cost of the equipment. For example, one vendor might charge more for the equipment, but another might charge more for delivery and setup.

Some mainstream computer vendors may offer to buy and install assistive technology as part of the package. This may not be a good idea unless the vendor has demonstrable experience with the technology in which you're interested.

It is sometimes possible to get good deals on used equipment. Used equipment may be available through garage sales, donations, eBay, or from other sources. Purchasing used equipment may be your only option for obtaining equipment that is no longer being manufactured. Be aware that the

124

Computer
Resources
for People
with
Disabilities

more complicated or extensive the equipment, the more likely it is that something may go wrong. For that reason, buying just a trackball on Ebay may have more satisfactory results than buying an entire computer system.

Regardless of the type of vendor you ultimately decide to work with, the most important thing is that you feel confident about the vendor's expertise and comfortable with their attitude. Does the vendor try to bluff responses to your questions, or are they honest enough to say, "I don't know" and willing to get back to you with a response later? Do they seem genuinely knowledgeable about the products, or do they seem to be parroting information? Are they willing to provide references on request? Are they patronizing?

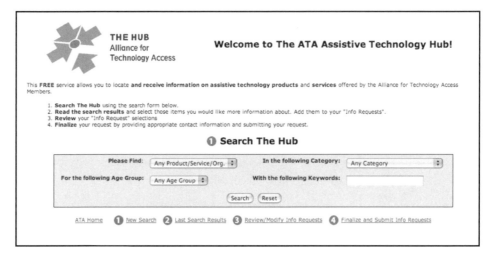

This is a sample web page from the ATA hub, an online database that assists people in finding vendor and product information.

Take the approach that both you and the vendor have a stake in establishing a long-term relationship. The vendor will want to keep you as an ongoing customer who can potentially refer others; you will want a reliable resource to contact for troubleshooting support and product-update information.

Worksheet 7A provides you with a beginning list of questions to ask potential vendors. As you start talking, you will likely develop additional questions of your own. Comparing answers from multiple vendors should help you make a final selection.

Worksheet 7A: Screening Questions for Potential Vendors

How much experience have you had selling the types of products I'm interested in? Are you an authorized dealer for these products?

_____

How do you stay up-to-date on new developments in both technology and rehabilitation?

_____

Do you carry professional liability insurance?

_____

In your experience, are the stated system requirements sufficient? If not, how should they be changed?

_____

_____

What is the warranty on your products? What is the process for getting products repaired or replaced? Do you provide loaner products while mine is being fixed?

_____

_____

What is your return policy for products that don't work properly? What is your policy for returning a product that works but doesn't meet my needs?

_____

_____

What type of equipment setup do you provide—e.g., will you bring the equipment to my office or home and get it working? Are there costs involved?

_____

_____

126

———

Computer
Resources
for People
with
Disabilities

Worksheet 7A: Screening Questions for Potential Vendors

What types of after-purchase (postsale) support do you provide? Are there costs involved?

_____

_____

Can you provide training on using my equipment if I need it? What are the costs involved?

_____

_____

Do you have any plans to discontinue or upgrade this product as new operating systems come along? Do you offer upgrade deals for current users?

_____

For services that you don't provide, are there other vendors you work with that you can recommend? Can you pass along their contact information if you have it?

_____

_____

Do you have a financing program available? What are the terms? Are there any situations (e.g., low-income buyer) where you provide discounts?

_____

_____

Can you provide the names of previous customers who use similar equipment and who I might contact as references?

_____

_____

Determine What Goes into the Budget

As mentioned earlier in the chapter, most people will have one of two budgeting scenarios: *flexible* (starting with the list of items you want to buy and creating a budget based upon their total cost) or *fixed* (starting with a set amount of money and purchasing items that add up to but do not surpass that amount). If your budget is flexible, you will start by listing the items you are considering and then totaling the cost. If your budget is fixed, you will start by listing the maximum amount of money you can spend and then deducting costs from this amount.

Regardless of whether you have a flexible or fixed budget, you may find yourself needing to prioritize acquisition of assistive-technology items. Try using the following criteria to help with this process:

Priority 1: Item is necessary in order for me to use the computer at all.

Example: Screen reader for an individual with no useable vision.

Priority 2: Item is not essential, but significantly contributes to my comfort or ease of use.

Example: Speech output in addition to a magnification program for someone who can usually see the screen with magnification alone.

Priority 3: Item is of interest for other reasons.

Example: Voice recognition programs for an individual who is satisfied with their typing ability.

You may then want to refine the budget, as necessary, by eliminating Priority 3 items, then eliminating one or more Priority 2 items.

Some budget items will occur more than once—e.g., monthly Internet-connection costs, annual service-plan charges, periodic costs to upgrade equipment. If you duplicate your initial budget worksheets and cross out lines for one-time purchases, you will be able to calculate these recurring costs as well.

Worksheets 7B and 7C provide you with a structure for determining your budget. Worksheet 7B is for people with a flexible budget, and Worksheet 7C is for people with a fixed budget. Use them not only for costs directly related to the computer but also for peripheral items such as ergonomic aids, furniture, and the like.

128

Computer
Resources
for People
with
Disabilities

Worksheet 7B: Flexible Budget

Item	Cost	Total
I. Total cost of basic computer configuration	_____	_____

Costs for Priority 1 item (duplicate this section for each Priority 1, 2, and 3 item)

Item	Cost	Total
Product cost	_____	
Shipping/handling/tax	_____	
Upgrade fee (optional; entitles you to a certain number of upgrades at reduced or no cost)	_____	
Installation charge	_____	
Training charge	_____	
Service-plan charge	_____	
Other charges	_____	
Subtotal A		_____

Computer upgrade costs necessary to use item:

Item	Cost	Total
Processor upgrade	_____	
Additional RAM	_____	
Sound card upgrade	_____	
Video card upgrade	_____	
Additional hard disk storage space	_____	
Additional removable media storage (e.g., ZIP drive and disks for storing large files)	_____	
Monitor upgrade	_____	
Additional peripherals (e.g., speakers)	_____	
Miscellaneous upgrade costs	_____	
Subtotal B		_____
Total for item (subtotal A + subtotal B)		_____

Item	Cost	Total
II. Total for all Priority 1 items	_____	_____
III. Total for all Priority 2 items	_____	_____
IV. Total for all Priority 3 items	_____	_____
V. Contingency fund for items not already covered**	_____	_____
TOTAL BUDGET (I + II + III + IV + V)	_____	

**(Suggested amount: 5% of I + II + III + IV)

Worksheet 7C: Fixed Budget

TOTAL BUDGET

Item	Cost	Balance*
I. Total cost of basic computer configuration		

Costs for Priority 1 item (duplicate this section for each Priority 1, 2, and 3 item)

Item	Cost
Product cost	
Shipping/handling/tax	
Upgrade fee (optional; entitles you to a certain number of upgrades at reduced or no cost)	
Installation charge	
Training charge	
Service-plan charge	
Other charges	
Subtotal A	

Computer upgrade costs necessary to use item:

Item	Cost
Processor upgrade	
Additional RAM	
Sound card upgrade	
Video card upgrade	
Additional hard disk storage space	
Additional removable media storage (e.g., ZIP drive and disks for storing large files)	
Monitor upgrade	
Additional peripherals (e.g., speakers)	
Miscellaneous upgrade costs	
Subtotal B	
Total for item (subtotal A + subtotal B)	

Item	Cost	Balance
II. Total for all Priority 1 items		
III. Total for all Priority 2 items		
IV. Total for all Priority 3 items		
V. Contingency fund for items not already covered**		
TOTAL BUDGET (I + II + III + IV + V)		
TOTAL REMAINING		

* Remaining budget (total budget minus cost of item)

**(Suggested amount: 5% of I + II + III + IV)

130

Computer
Resources
for People
with
Disabilities

How Life Situations Impact Budgeting for and Buying Technology

Outlined below are considerations that may affect the processes of budgeting for and buying technology at different life stages.

Preschool

Because the technology needs of preschool students are limited and specific, it is particularly important to find a vendor with whom you feel comfortable. Ask about the vendor's experience in providing equipment to very young children, and ask what implementation strategies have and have not worked. A helpful strategy will be to find someone who can appropriately meet your current needs and then go back to that same person as your child's needs change.

K–12 (Public or Private)

It is almost impossible to assume that what works for a child in first grade will still be effective by the time she reaches sixth grade. There are simply too many variables, including school standards for what hardware and software is used, and changes to the child's growing body. It is therefore important, regardless of the funding source, that some anticipation of the need for upgraded equipment be included in a long-term budget.

Higher Education

Colleges and universities often provide specifications for equipment that students should bring with them—for example, specifications addressing compatibility with campus computing systems or class work requirements. As early in the process as possible, you should ask for a list of these specifications and factor them into the budget.

Transition from School to Work/In the Workplace

Employers will naturally be skeptical about spending more money on assistive technology than they feel they have to. Even if you will not be funding the equipment purchase yourself, it may be helpful to go through the processes outlined in this chapter and provide the information to your employer. This will provide both of you with a clear picture of the costs of your accommodation. Doing so is especially important if the computers already owned by the employer are insufficient to run the equipment you need.

Back to Work (Reentry)

Third-party funding sources (e.g., state departments of rehabilitation) often work primarily with "approved" vendors and may need significant justification to purchase equipment from a nonapproved vendor. Check with your counselor to see who their approved vendors are and what their policies are on buying equipment from other vendors.

At Home/Daily Living

Don't hesitate to get input on both vendor selection and budgeting from friends, family, and roommates, particularly if they will be using the computer as well. They are likely to provide a fresh perspective, as well as contribute information about their own experiences.

Accessing Technology in the Community

If you are going to be purchasing your own technology, you will be less reliant on the accessibility of publicly available workstations. However, you will still need to make sure your equipment works with services provided by businesses and organizations with which you need to interact. For example, will your screen reading software work effectively with your local library's website? Will your TTY interface with your bank's voice-mail system? If you are having difficulty, contact the business or organization and ask what its current or anticipated solutions might be. Then put any additional system requirements (e.g., a dedicated Internet connection) into your budget.

Injury, Illness

If you have only a short-term need for assistive technology, the trial period provided by demonstration software may be sufficient for your needs. If it isn't, you may need to weigh the costs of acquiring and learning to use some assistive technologies against common limitations in using free or low-cost solutions. For example, if you have a broken wrist that is expected to heal completely, purchasing and learning to use a one-handed keyboard may be an option. However, you can also activate the built-in sticky-key control-panel option on your current computer and continue using your standard keyboard until the wrist heals.

Aging

Many of the natural effects and conditions associated with aging are unstable; they may worsen or improve over time or from day to day. The best solution is to pick assistive technology that permits flexible settings and,

132

—

Computer
Resources
for People
with
Disabilities

optimally, allows those settings to be saved as preferences that can be accessed at will. If one access solution doesn't consistently meet your needs, however, you may need to budget for the acquisition of multiple solutions to be used in combination or at different times. Make sure that these multiple technologies work well together; even products from the same company may not be fully compatible.

Up and Running

How Will I Set Up My Equipment and Learn to Use It?

Dennis R. Welton, manager of instructional services/rehabilitation engineer, the STAR Center, Jackson, Tennessee

The Big Picture: Where You Are in Your AT Planning Process

The boxes have been delivered. You anticipate using your new technology as soon as possible. Now that you have your equipment, the next step is to get it set up and running. We think you will find this part of your journey to be the most fun. Once you have acquired the right computer and/or assistive-technology system, much of the pressure is off, and you can begin enjoying and working with your new system.

In this chapter we focus on providing the tools necessary to get you up and running in almost no time with your new equipment. You can then pursue the fulfillment of your original goals and be free to experiment, improvise, and discover other uses for your system. Before we plunge in, reflect on other suggestions provided in this book that may directly influence the way you approach this phase. Whether you enter the process at this stage or have been reading and completing the worksheets in other chapters of the book, consider the following:

- Have you identified who can assist you with the setup and training processes and how to build a team of support? Taking these steps first may make this stage easier for you.

- Have you budgeted for technical support, if needed?

Useful Preparation

Before you begin to set up your equipment—possibly even before your new equipment arrives—take some time to prepare for the new arrival. Careful

134

Computer
Resources
for People
with
Disabilities

preparation will minimize delays and frustrations in the setup of your new equipment. The suggestions outlined below should help with this step:

- Refer to Worksheet 8A, "Getting Ready to Install Your New System." You may wish to photocopy it so you can keep track of your process and take notes.

- Be aware that virtually every piece of equipment and all of the more expensive software programs contain serial numbers. Record your serial numbers and store them in a safe place. Also, keep a copy posted near your computer in case you need to contact technical support about a particular product.

- Fill out the warranty and/or registration cards and send them in. These register you as a customer and establish a purchase date. Most warranties cover products for one year from the date of purchase.

  - Registering your product may put you on the manufacturer's mailing list to receive information regarding updates or recalls. Some warranty cards register you for technical support services.

  - Keep a copy of the cards in case you encounter problems later. It's also a good idea to keep the original packaging in case you need to return products or have them serviced. This is especially true of high-cost devices, such as computers, augmentative or alternative communication devices, and environmental-control units.

- Make sure you have an accessible work space set aside for the new equipment. The area should be clear of any obstructions so that there is enough room for your desk or workstation.

- Make sure that there are enough power outlets and telephone jacks (for a modem) in your work space.

- If you are connecting a computer to a broadband connection for Internet access (e.g., cable or DSL), make sure that your work space and workstation have enough space to accommodate the extra equipment and cabling.

- Make sure that you have enough space to set up your assistive-technology devices—especially if you have large pieces, such as a closed-circuit TV, a Braille printer, etc.

- Read the installation information. Before you begin installing any type of equipment, always read the manual first, especially if it says "Read Me First" in large red letters.

- If you have some knowledge of computers, you may want to go to the "quick start" portion of the manual to get your basic computer system up and running.

- Have the manual available in case you run into something you don't understand or have questions during the setup.

- If you are a beginner, do yourself a favor and read through the manual step-by-step. Despite reputations to the contrary, most manuals are now fairly easy to follow, jargon-free, and helpful to people who want to start using their equipment quickly.

• Read the manuals for your assistive devices thoroughly. Spending a little more time at the beginning to make sure everything is set up correctly could save you from having to go back and troubleshoot later.

- You may come across information about something that is easier to set up/configure before you complete the installation of other parts of the complete system, including the computer.

136

Computer
Resources
for People
with
Disabilities

Worksheet 8A: Getting Ready
to Install Your New System

Step 1: What Do I Have on Hand?

Equipment inventory (refer to packing list/invoice)

Device _____

Cables _____

	What else is needed?	**Is it on hand?**
Power cord/supply	_____	_____
Accessories	_____	_____
Monitor	_____	_____
Keyboard	_____	_____
Mouse	_____	_____
Printer	_____	_____
Surge protector	_____	_____
Other: _____	_____	_____
Other: _____	_____	_____
Other: _____	_____	_____

Is my workstation set up to accommodate the device? _____

Step 2: Where Do I Plan to Locate the Equipment?

Planned location: _____

	Current dimensions	**Needed dimensions:**
Depth	_____ (inches)	_____
Length	_____ (inches)	_____
Width	_____ (inches)	_____

Power outlets:

Number of power outlets I have? _____

Number I need? _____

Phone jack: _____

Telephone jacks present? _____

Do they meet my requirements? _____

Step 3: Additional Software and Materials

What software do I have/need?	**Have**	**Need**
Operating system (e.g., Windows)	_____	_____
Antivirus software	_____	_____
Office productivity package (e.g., Microsoft Office)	_____	_____
Internet (e.g., AOL, MSN)	_____	_____
Other: _____	_____	_____
Other: _____	_____	_____

What materials/accessories do I have/need?

Instruction manual:	_____	_____
Additional information from the vendor	_____	_____
Other: _____	_____	_____

Step 4: Tools

What tools do I have/need for setup?

Screwdriver?	_____	_____
Allen wrench?	_____	_____
Socket driver and sockets?	_____	_____
Hammer?	_____	_____
Other: _____	_____	_____

Step 5: Additional Help

Do I need any additional help with setup?

Yes _____   No _____

If yes, contact appropriate agencies.

138

Computer
Resources
for People
with
Disabilities

Steps to Consider

What if you cannot physically handle your computer or if you feel uncomfortable setting it up or connecting the assistive devices? Some computer stores will set up the computer in your home for a nominal fee if you purchased the machine from them. If you bought your computer by mail order, however, you will need to find another source of help.

Determining Who Can Help

Computer clubs and user groups can be excellent resources, as they are filled with people who enjoy setting up computer systems and who may be happy to show off their skills. For the most part, they will know conventional technology but may or may not be able to help you figure out the assistive technology.

You might contact the assistive-technology vendor about setup support. The vendor may have other customers who would be interested in providing some assistance to you.

Additionally, you may want to develop a relationship with your local vocational-rehabilitation (VR) office or career center, if you have not already done so. As discussed in earlier chapters, these agencies can help with the purchasing of equipment. In addition, they are good sources of assistance when it comes to setting up your equipment and getting training for the use of all of your devices. The VR agency may refer you to a local rehabilitation center, such as an ATA-affiliated center, that can assist you in the setup of your system.

Whatever your needs are, or if you have any doubts about your ability to set up your system, make sure these are addressed prior to installing the equipment.

Setting Up Your Equipment

The manuals that came with your computer and assistive devices contain diagrams that show how to hook up everything. Many systems have matching icons on the cables and hardware to make connections easier. Most equipment cables now have connectors that can be tightened by hand, although some require an ordinary screwdriver. As you begin to set up your equipment, approach it using the following three-stage method, roughly outlined in Worksheet 8A:

Stage 1—Unpacking the Device

1. Inventory the contents. Compare them to the packing list.

2. Check for broken or damaged parts.

3. Check for all needed parts and components.

4. Contact the vendor if any parts are broken, damaged, or missing.

Stage 2—Preparing the Workstation and Work Space

Do you have to assemble your workstation?

Yes _____   No _____ (skip to Stage 3 below)

Assemble your workstation:

1. Inventory the parts.

2. Obtain the necessary tools (see instructions that came with workstation).

3. Contact vendor if any parts are missing or damaged.

4. Remove any nonessential items from and around your workstation.

5. Clean surface(s) of workstation.

Stage 3—Putting the System Together

1. Refer to the instructions that came with the device. Look at the "quick start" guide and/or setup guides.

2. Connect the parts of the device together.

Note the following important points:

- If you are working with a system that includes a computer, it is imperative that you first get the computer running with its basic component parts. Once the computer system works, you can add your assistive-technology pieces one at a time.

- After you install each piece of assistive technology, make sure to verify that it is working without errors or other problems before moving on to the installation of the next piece.

- If you have one or more pieces of assistive technology that have text-to-speech capability, make sure to do some extra research into the installation for each one. Some programs need to be installed before others of the same type or else they will not work.

Once you have your system up and running, it's time to develop proficiency with your technology. The same agencies that help with setup can also assist you in obtaining training on your new equipment.

140

Computer
Resources
for People
with
Disabilities

Taking Environmental Considerations into Account

As you establish a home for your equipment, keep in mind that some environments are unfriendly to computers and other technology.

- Avoid locations that are too hot or cold, that are too dusty, or that have the potential to be moist. Placement too close to a window may create temperature-control problems and may interfere with the visibility of the monitor because of glare.

- Make sure there is plenty of space for the CPU and the cables you connect; do not push the CPU against a wall or enclose it in a tight space. E-mail and Internet access will require you to locate your equipment near a telephone outlet or to use a long telephone cord.

- Keep your system away from moisture—such as drinks and high humidity—that can affect the tiny circuits of the computer. If necessary, use a moisture guard (a thin, plastic keyboard cover that provides extra protection (for more information see "Keyboard Additions" in Part II)).

- Magnetic fields create problems. Keep all magnets away from the computer. Some common sources of magnetic fields are speakers, telephones, radios, refrigerator magnets, and paper clips that have become magnetized by a paper-clip dispenser.

- Static electricity may be annoying to you, but it is dangerous for your computer. If you have problems with static electricity, purchase a grounding strip that allows static electricity to be harmlessly eliminated. Grounding strips are available in most hardware stores.

- Avoid smoke of any kind around the computer, as it can damage the disk drives and circuits. Keep the computer away from your stove or oven, where fumes from burning food can enter your computer and cause problems. This is especially true of self-cleaning ovens.

- To avoid damage to any of the components, turn your computer off before hooking up or unhooking any devices.

- Store individual floppy disks with caution. Magnetic fields can erase disk information. Storing disks in a box, away from extreme temperatures, will help ensure their safety. Don't bend diskettes or place heavy objects on them. The metal clip on 3.5-inch disks can become bent or jammed if not handled carefully. You can buy inexpensive disk holders at any computer store.

- Store individual CD-ROM discs in either a CD-ROM case with individual pockets for your discs or in their jewel cases. This will reduce the chance that they will become damaged or unreadable.

Positioning the Components of Your System

The science of ergonomics focuses on the effects of computer use on the human body. It is important that you take preventive measures to avoid problems from the effects of computer use on your body. Take frequent breaks from the computer. Doing so is good for the body, eyes, and mind.

Make your computer setup as comfortable as possible. Easy access and comfort are the top priorities. The table surface on which you put the computer should be low enough so that when you sit you are looking down slightly at the monitor. If you are using a standard keyboard and mouse, your hands should rest comfortably on the desk and keyboard. Wrist rests and arm supports can help make your computing environment more healthful and comfortable.

If the computer must accommodate several different users or must be moved around between home, school, and work, use adjustable-height tables and tables on wheels. For very young users, consider using a table close to the ground, where children can stand to work on the computer or sit on small chairs. Office-furniture stores and catalogs are sources for these types of tables and other computer furniture. Furniture does not have to be expensive, but it needs to work well for you. Also, be sure to allot an adequate amount of tabletop or desk space, since computers and assistive devices take up a fair amount of space.

Monitors can be placed on top of or alongside the CPU. We have even seen monitors placed on the floor to provide access to young children. If more than one person or another person with a physical disability will be using the computer, consider a floating monitor arm. This is a mechanical arm that connects to a table and allows the monitor to move up, down, in, and out with ease, thus allowing people to change positions during the day and move the monitor into a position for best access.

Keyboard placement is also adjustable; place the keyboard and other input devices where they can be used comfortably.

Be creative. It is not necessary to set up your computer to look like an ad in the Sunday paper. Some—but not all—CPUs can be turned on their sides. You can put the CPU on the floor or in another place to provide easier access to the disk drive. There are even CPU holders that are designed to mount the CPU under or to the side of your desk while still keeping it off of the ground. Keyboards can be mounted on trays, angled, or padded to fit the user.

142

———

Computer
Resources
for People
with
Disabilities

Powering Up

Rather than plugging your computer directly into the wall, we recommend using a power strip, which comes in many styles and prices. Some have filters, and some provide protection against power surges or significant current fluctuations. Unless you have a special requirement or a power problem in your area, a simple power strip with a surge protector should meet your needs inexpensively. While a basic power strip may be effective, it is well worth the extra $5 to $10 to get a surge protector that offers a guarantee. The manufacturers of surge protectors guarantee that they will replace the electronic equipment that is plugged into their strip if it is damaged by a power surge or lightning strike.

If you cannot activate the small toggle on the power strip, there are a number of alternative ways to get electricity to the power strip. There are power modules that can be activated by a switch and mounted anywhere. A tread switch is an on/off switch that can be activated by rolling a wheelchair across it. Many solutions can be individualized to meet your needs. For these types of setups you may want to consult with a rehabilitation engineer or other assistive-technology practitioner (ATP) to assist in determining what will best work for you.

If, when you press the switch on the power strip, it whirs and beeps and you get a DOS prompt, a Windows menu, or a "happy Mac" icon, you may want to let out a cheer. You have successfully powered up!

Troubleshooting

If, however, you press the switch and nothing happens, you need to investigate or troubleshoot the problem. Your problem could be something simple, such as a loose plug or cable, or something more technical, such as a conflict among special utility programs within your system. If you suspect the latter, it's time to make some phone calls. Before you call, however, always check all your cable connections!

If you bought the equipment at a local computer store, call them first. You might also call the vendor of your assistive technology if it seems to be a problem that came about when a particular piece of AT was attached to the system. You can also try the toll-free support number that came with your computer. All major companies have support-staff members who answer questions and troubleshoot problems. But don't expect them to know anything about your assistive technology.

When making these types of troubleshooting calls, have the following on hand:

1. The model number of each piece of equipment.

2. The version of the operating system you are running (e.g., Windows 98, Windows ME, Windows XP, Macintosh OSX, etc.)

3. If possible, have your computer turned on and near the telephone so you can test the suggestions offered.

If you can't resolve the problem, call on your support team. Remember, support team members are there to help. Refer to the next chapter for more possibilities for troubleshooting any problems you have with your system.

Once you get started, we recommend you use your computer as much as possible during the warranty period. If anything is going to go wrong with the machinery, it will most likely happen during this period. Also, you will become comfortable with your new tools more quickly if you spend concentrated time using them right from the beginning.

Learning and Training

Personal computing is in some ways getting more intuitive. You can learn a great deal on your own or with the help of a friend or two and by taking some time to play with the computer.

Begin by going through the material you received with the computer. Many computer companies include good step-by-step tutorials on disk, which cover using the mouse, opening and closing files, saving data, printing, and other basic skills.

When it comes to learning software, do not underestimate your ability to train yourself. Many technology users are self-trained and enjoyed every minute of the process. Everything you buy will come with instructions, and many software programs have on-disk tutorials. If you purchased a computer with some software already installed, get to know those programs first. There is nothing like learning to use the mouse by playing a few hundred games of solitaire. Install one program at a time and learn how to use it before moving to the next program on your list. This way, installing your software doesn't become overwhelming. As your confidence builds, you will look forward to experimenting with the next piece of software.

A number of training videotapes and audiotapes with disk activities for popular software titles are available, as is a growing assortment of introductory books on the major computer systems. All are available in local book and computer stores, at the library, and through Internet booksellers. Check with your sources for their favorite titles.

Whenever you are experimenting or troubleshooting a problem, do one thing at a time and keep track of what you did. If you make a mistake, it will be easier to fix. If you get it right, you'll know what you did and be able to do it again.

144

Computer
Resources
for People
with
Disabilities

Don't be afraid to try things. Many new computer users believe they can bring about disaster by pressing the wrong key or making the wrong choice at the wrong time. You really can't blow up a computer by pressing the wrong key. Disasters can be avoided fairly easily. Here are a few suggestions to help eliminate both the fears and the disasters:

- Experiment. Once you are in a program and your work is saved, look around. Make choices, push buttons, pull down the menus. You usually can't do much harm if you have saved your data. And you can always reload the program if something really goes wrong.

- Save your work. Learn how to save your work before you learn how to do anything else. Get into the habit of saving your work on a hard disk or on a diskette. Save often. Save compulsively. In the case of a power failure or a system error, you will lose anything you haven't saved to disk.

- A system error—also known as a crash—happens to everyone at one time or another, and it simply means there is a temporary problem with your operating system. The treatment for a crash is to turn off your computer and restart—or reboot—your computer. If the problem persists, seek advice.

- Back up your work. Keep copies of your work and your applications (your software programs) on disks, and store them in a safe place. Making a copy of your data can save you a great deal of time and frustration if anything happens to the hard disk or an individual disk.

Obtaining Additional Support

There are times and situations that call for a more structured approach to learning computing. Everyone has his or her own learning style, and awareness of your own style should guide you in selecting a teaching method or instructor to meet your needs. Private teachers can tailor their approach to match your style and preferred pace. Check your community resources and contacts for referrals.

There are quite a few options for learning how to use conventional technologies. Resources such as the following typically offer beginning, intermediate, and advanced classes:

- community colleges

- computer user groups

- adult-education programs of local school districts

- computer stores

- copying service centers

Often overlooked places to obtain training include local community technology centers (CTCs) and local libraries. Classes usually focus on a particular type of computer or on a particular software application, such as a word processing or spreadsheet program. Many classes are available to help you get started on the Internet or to teach you how to design web pages. Enrollment fees are usually modest.

Question the suppliers of training as you would vendors of equipment and software. Ask if you can preview sessions or visit the location, and learn what you can about follow-up or ongoing support. Accessibility of the training site and the equipment might be concerns for you. If you need assistive devices to access their computer systems, you will probably need to bring them to participate in the class. Be aware that the instructor will be teaching the class how to use a keyboard and a mouse and will probably know little about how to assist you with your adaptive devices.

Learning to Use Your Assistive Technology

Finding training in how to use assistive technologies is more complex. As we mentioned in the chapter on budgeting, it is important during your planning to set money aside for training. When comparing prices, ask vendors if they provide training. This may explain why one vendor charges more money for a certain product than a competitor. Factor in what it would take to get training elsewhere if it's not included in the price of the product. Vendors that don't offer training may be able to point you toward an individual or organization in your area that has purchased the same device. Many people who have mastered a device themselves are happy to share their expertise. In addition, private tutors and consultants can help people learn how to use adaptive equipment.

Using assistive technology successfully takes time and practice, since you are learning to use it in addition to learning how to use the basic computer and programs. It may be helpful to work with someone experienced with the particular components you have on your computer, whether it is a screen reader for navigation, an alternative input device, or some other assistive technology. A support person who can offer strategies for learning to operate your system will be invaluable in guiding you through the steep learning curve that may be involved, saving you time and frustration in the long run. Whether you go it alone or use support, remember the perseverance it took to obtain the tools, and apply that same persistence to the process of learning to use your new system.

146

Computer
Resources
for People
with
Disabilities

Some assistive-technology centers, community colleges, and other community-based programs offer classes in using assistive technology. Some community colleges—in California, for example—do have such courses and provide accessible computer labs. However, you may need to enroll as a student in order to take advantage of these classes.

If your community does not offer these opportunities, ask for them. Talk to people who offer educational programs about what it would take to make the existing program accessible and how you can assist them in making it work. The ultimate goal should not be to set up separate learning environments, but rather to make existing ones accessible.

Learning to use your assistive technology, along with the other components of your system, is a critical step in your process. If you do not learn how to effectively use your equipment—especially the assistive technology—the possibility of "abandoning" your system greatly increases. This is due to the extreme frustration that results from the inability to work the equipment. For this reason, make sure that you receive adequate training on your system. When in training, do not be afraid to ask questions or ask for clarification about particular points or features of the technology. The more you know about your technology, the better you will be at using it and the better you will be at knowing when it is not operating correctly and needs someone to look at it.

Building Up Your Support Network

Taking advantage of continuing-education opportunities in your community can be one of the most beneficial moves you will make to learn new skills and to network with others in your community. Many universities and teachers colleges offer courses in the use of technology for students with disabilities. In some cases, these courses are required for degree candidates in special education. University extension programs and community-based organizations also offer opportunities for teachers to learn about assistive technology and to receive continuing-education units (CEUs) in the process.

Computer conferences are conducted around the country. In addition to opportunities to see and test new products, they often offer training on various products, especially in classroom and clinical settings. These are great opportunities for you to meet others who are using the same type of technology as you are and who will have additional ideas and information about using the technology. Individuals you meet at conferences can become part of your extended circle of support, offering you both perspective and experience with the technology.

Reflect on ways the technology can support your strengths and minimize your weaknesses. This will help you to better utilize your new system and maximize the assistance it can provide you. The better you understand your equipment, the better you will become at using it.

How Life Situations Impact the Setup and Use of Your Equipment

The things you need to consider will vary according to your life situation and environment. Below are lists of life stage–specific suggestions and considerations that should help you find solutions.

Preschool

For parents, teachers, or rehabilitation professionals setting up a system for a young child:

- Keep in mind the needs of the child(ren) who will be using the system.

- Focus on making the system as simple and user-friendly as possible.

- Make the system as error-free as it can be.

- If more than one child uses the system, make sure that the setup is easily modified to reflect the different needs of the children who will be using it. Long delays in setup will cause loss of valuable working time and can trigger frustration on the part of the child.

- Make sure that the parent and any other professionals are adequately trained on the use of the system—both conventional and AT. Inadequate training will cause frustration and decreased productivity on the part of both the child(ren) and the parent or other professional(s) working with them.

K–12 (Public or Private)

For teachers, rehabilitation counselors, and other professionals setting up a system for a child in grades K–12:

- Keep in mind the needs of the child(ren) who will be using the system, as well as the age group for which it will be set up.

- Make sure that access technologies are in place, are working, and are easily changed by any staff working with the system.

- Before the child is introduced to the system, make sure that all professionals working with the system are trained in the use of all of its parts.

148

Computer
Resources
for People
with
Disabilities

- Keep the school system's information technology (IT) team informed about all assistive technology to be used on the system. Offer training on all such technology to IT staff. Doing so will help to reduce any stress or friction between the teacher, the parent, and the school IT team. It will also create support for the technology within the school.

For parents setting up a system for their child who is enrolled in K–12 education:

- Make sure that the setup you have at home works with the system at school.

- Make sure that you keep communication open between yourself and school personnel about the system and about any needs or ideas that you may identify while working with your child at home.

Higher Education

- Do you have enough space and enough power outlets for all of your equipment?

- Do you have a roommate(s) who will be sharing your space?

- Will they be sharing your equipment? If so, set some ground rules on equipment use so that your assistive technology is always available for your use.

Transition from School to Work

- Reestablish or expand your support network.

- Who will be your technical support for any problems you encounter on the job?

- Will your system from school make the transition with you to the job, or will new equipment be provided?

- If new equipment is needed, make sure you are in contact with your VR counselor (if you have one) to help identify your needs at work.

In the Workplace

- Check how much space you will have for your equipment.

- Do you need to contact the employer's IT staff to assist you in setup?

- Do you need any additional equipment in order for you to perform your job duties?

Back to Work (Reentry)

- Do you need to upgrade your equipment to meet the needs of the job?

- Do you need to contact the employer's IT staff to assist in setup?

- Do you need any additional equipment to perform your job duties?

At Home/Daily Living

- Is there a place in your home that is adequate and safe for your equipment?

- Make sure that you get adequate training for everyone involved in the use of the system.

- Develop a support network. Doing so is essential to long-term success and trouble-free operation.

In the Community

- Is the system configured for use in the community (i.e., are there communication page-sets on your AAC device for community activities)?

- Do not attempt to install all assistive-technology products on one computer if you are working in a public setting, such as in a community technology center, a campus lab, or a public library. Doing so will often result in conflicts. It also limits the availability of that computer.

Injury and Illness

- As a result of an injury or illness, have any of the following changed:

  - Your access method?

  - Your ability to use your equipment?

- As a result of any changes to your access, do you:

  - Need additional training on your equipment?

  - Need additional equipment?

Chapter 9

Repairs and Upgrades

How Do I Keep My Technology Working for Me?

Nancy Story, assistive-technology practitioner, Technology Resource Solutions for People, Salina, Kansas

Janice Fouard, assistive technology and agricultural specialist, Technology Resource Solutions for People, Salina, Kansas

Kathy Reed, assistive technology practitioner, Technology Resource Solutions for People, Salina, Kansas

The Big Picture: Where You Are in Your AT Planning Process

In this chapter we focus on strategies for dealing with breakdowns and upgrades. First, reflect on other material you've encountered in this book that may directly influence the way you approach this phase. Whether you enter the process at this stage or have been reading and working through other chapters in the book, consider the following:

- **Know your funding strategies.** Have you developed a funding strategy to pay for the technology? Do you have money set aside for repairs and upgrades? (Refer to Chapter 6 for information on funding strategies.)

- **Determine your "people" resources and build a team of support.** Have you determined who can assist you through the process of upgrading or selecting new software or peripherals? (Refer to Chapter 3 for specific information on how to tap into your "people" resources and obtain both support and knowledge.)

- **Assess your technology needs and set your goals.** Are you clear about what you want to accomplish with the support of technology? Have new technologies become available since your initial purchase? Have your skills or access needs changed? (Refer to Chapter 2 for suggestions on how to assess your needs and set your goals.)

- **Know what equipment you want to purchase.** Have you selected the types of equipment you want and talked with vendors? Have you compared the cost of repairing old versus buying new equipment? (Refer to Chapter 4 for information on selecting equipment.)

- **Determine your training needs.** Have you identified what further training you may need in order to be able to use your equipment? This includes training in assistive technology, computer basics, and the use of any new software or peripherals that have been added to your system. (Refer to Chapter 8 for information on how to determine your training needs and options.)

Useful Preparation

To help you organize the steps involved in deciding on and implementing repairs and upgrades, we have provided worksheets throughout this chapter. You may wish to photocopy them so you can keep track of your process and take notes. Before you make any decisions about spending money on repairs and upgrades, take note of these useful pointers:

- Know as much as possible about your equipment's specifications.

- Have a clear picture of what equipment problems are occurring.

- Have pertinent manuals, software, and CDs handy and organized.

Steps to Consider

The remainder of the chapter will guide you through the details of making decisions about repairs and upgrades by helping you answer the following questions:

- What, specifically, needs to be upgraded or repaired?

- What are my current and long-term technology needs?

- What vendor, group, or individual will I use for technical support?

- What do I need to know before I turn to outside support?

The following story illustrates both the challenges and rewards of getting technology to work as well as how it is a continuous effort that takes a lot of support.

My name is *Dan*. I sustained a head injury at the age of 32. Now I am 44. My interest in computers began when I was in a rehabilitation program

152

Computer
Resources
for People
with
Disabilities

in Colorado. While working on budgets, I realized a computer could really help me. I went to the computer lab every day, working on budgets and to-do lists. Staff told me they wished others were as motivated as I was. Learning the computer held my interest and helped me accomplish my goals.

When I moved back to Salina, Kansas, people began telling me of all the interesting things on the Internet. I began to hear that people could sell items online, and I decided that I would like to sell antiques online. Because of the way I talk, my disability, my use of the wheelchair, and the presence of curbs and other physical barriers, I had run into discrimination when doing business face-to-face with antique dealers. I wouldn't have that problem online!

The process took three years. It was not easy. I was faced with finding funds to get equipment. I also had to cope with technology breakdowns and replacements that were very challenging. It seemed that every time I turned around, another part of my system needed fixing!

I was able to get ideas from the staff at my local assistive-technology center, from a computer vendor, and from my family. Their input made the process, although still difficult, more manageable.

On the positive side, I have been able to accomplish many of my goals using technology. I recently purchased a digital camera, so I now include pictures of the items listed for sale online. Technology will always change, and I will need to keep pace, so there isn't an end to my story. It is a story that will go on for 30 or 40 more years.

How to Find Technical Support

You may be your own technical support. If that's the case, when you experience a computer problem, relax and rethink. Power down, shut off, and reboot your equipment—and yourself. Give yourself time to think through simple troubleshooting options. Sometimes stepping away from the problem for half an hour—or even for a day or two, if you have the time—and then coming back to it later leads to fresh ideas and a lower frustration level. If your ideas fail to solve the problem, then it may be time to contact outside support.

Consider your options for outside technical support. Your financial resources or the extent of the problem may dictate whom you will contact. A few options are listed below:

- **Knowledgeable student.** Your local school system, technical schools, and colleges may have students who need a project or who simply enjoy the challenge of working with various computer users.

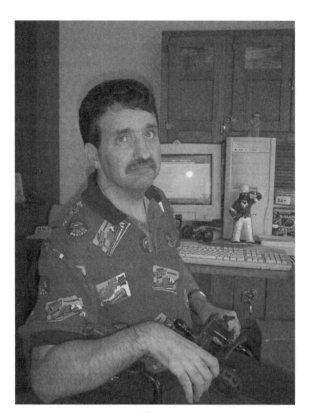

Dan

- **Family member, friend, or neighbor.** Someone you know may be knowledgeable enough to fix the problem, or they may assist you in getting through the process.

- **Yellow Pages; look under "computer repair."** On the other hand, if you are having problems with specialized adaptive equipment, you may need to call the original vendor.

- **Company or vendor who sold you the equipment.** Read this chapter to be prepared to work with the vendor.

- **Vendor's technical-support phone line, website, or manual.** In addition to or in lieu of a phone conversation, explore the different methods a vendor offers for troubleshooting. If you can use the Internet, try the vendor's website for solutions. Look through the manual, especially the "troubleshooting" section.

- **Technology-access centers and community technology centers (CTCs).** Locate your local technology-access center. It may be an Alliance for Technology Access (ATA) site or another local program. Such centers are often a good connection to a large network of

154

Computer
Resources
for People
with
Disabilities

individuals with disabilities, parents, educators, friends, and vendors who are glad to share their expertise.

- **Technical assistance projects.** Each state's method of providing technical assistance is unique. By contacting the lead office in your state, you can obtain information about their range of services and other helpful referral information.

What to Know Before You Call for Help

Define your problem. It may be simple or complicated. Is an obvious problem being overlooked? Is there something you can do before calling outside support? Worksheet 9A, "Problem-Solving Checklist," contains ideas for the first steps to consider. Later, if you decide to contact support, you will have already gathered key information that may save you time and money.

Manuals offer a great deal of information, but you will occasionally encounter a difficulty or want to perform a task you cannot find described in the manual. Fortunately, most software and hardware companies have technical-support people on staff who work every day to make sure customers are getting the most from their purchase. Depending on the severity of the problem, the vendor or individual who sold you the equipment may be the first person you should consider contacting.

Vendors that provide a full range of support may charge a little more for their products. You may encounter a situation in which one vendor offers a better price, while another provides better service. Ongoing vendor support can be crucial, and we recommend dealing with vendors that provide good support even if they charge more for the same products than a competitor that offers little or no support. Before contacting a vendor for technical support, complete Worksheet 9B in order to gather the needed information about your system.

Problem	Notes
Will the computer start?	
If NO, ask yourself the following questions:	
☐ Is the computer plugged into a power strip or outlet?	
☐ Is the power cord plugged in tightly at both ends?	
☐ If the computer is plugged into a power strip, is the power strip on?	
☐ Does the problem happen at the same place in the start-up sequence every time? If it does, what is on the screen when the problem occurs?	
☐ Are you getting an error message? If so, write the message in the Notes area.	
Is it just the monitor that is not working?	
If YES, ask yourself the following questions:	
☐ Is it turned on? Is the monitor's indicator light on, if it has one?	
☐ Is the power cord plugged in tightly at both ends?	
Is the problem that the mouse, keyboard, printer, or items such as an adaptive keyboard are not working?	
If YES, ask yourself the following questions:	
☐ Are the cords plugged into the CPU tightly?	
☐ Have you tried restarting the computer?	
☐ Have you tried reinstalling any special software that supports the peripheral equipment (such as a printer driver)?	

156

Computer
Resources
for People
with
Disabilities

<u>**Worksheet 9A:** Problem-Solving Checklist (cont'd.)</u>

Problem	Notes
Are the problems occurring only in a specific software program?	
☐ Was it working before? If so, has anything changed (e.g., have you installed new software, thrown away some files, etc.)?	
☐ Have you turned off all power to the computer, waited a few minutes, and restarted?	
☐ Are you getting an error message? If so, write the message in the Notes area.	

What events led to the problem? Write down what you know about the problem.

Other Notes

Worksheet 9B: Information You Need Before You Call the Vendor

Information to gather:

Completed problem-solving checklist _____

Vendor phone numbers _____

Does the vendor have a toll-free number? _____

Warranty information and date of purchase

_____

_____

Serial and model numbers of computer and assistive-technology products

_____

_____

_____

Original software with corresponding manuals and registration numbers

_____

_____

_____

_____

_____

Processor speed of your computer _____

RAM, or memory, of your computer _____

Questions to ask:

Is my warranty still in effect? _____

Is there a charge for technical assistance? _____

If my equipment needs to be sent in, is there a loan of similar equipment available? _____

If I send in the equipment, how long will it be before it is returned?

_____

158

Computer
Resources
for People
with
Disabilities

What to Know Before You Upgrade

You may have noticed that upgrading occurs on two levels: The technology is advancing, and so are you. You may have started out in awe of what technology could do, but now, as a more sophisticated user, you have higher expectations and want the technology to do more for you.

No matter which system and adaptation you purchase, you will probably want to add additional hardware or peripherals at some point. Think about what you need the device to do now and in the future. The following steps will help guide you through the process of upgrading or dealing with breakdowns:

- **How old is the device, and can it be upgraded?** Keep all of the documentation that came with your system. A simple call to the vendor may answer your questions about upgrading the system.

- **What are the specifications for the programs and peripherals you want?** If you need specialized software, such as voice recognition or screen reading programs, be aware of the specifications the vendor suggests for running the program. These specifications are printed on the software package; alternatively, they can be found by calling the vendor or checking the vendor's website. The following are the sorts of questions you will want to have answers to:

  - How much memory is needed for this software?

  - What processor speed is recommended?

  - Is there adequate space on the hard drive?

  - Would the software benefit from a larger monitor?

  - Is the software compatible with your current operating system (Windows 98, Windows 2000, Windows XP, or Macintosh)?

  - If there is a compatibility issue between the software you are considering and your system, is a patch available from the vendor?

If you want to upgrade components of your computer, it is helpful to know the specifications of your system. All computers have a ceiling beyond which you cannot add components, memory, and the like; a dealer can tell you what limits are required for upgrading your computer. Depending on the upgrade, it may be less expensive in the long run to replace the original system. Ask the following questions:

- **How are future upgrades handled?**

- **What costs and ordering procedures will be involved when upgrades are released?** Registered users of a product or service will often be able to receive upgrades with little effort or cost. However, dramatically improved software products may require an upgrade fee of $50 to $100 or more.

- **Does the vendor offer a service agreement that would cover the next three or more upgrades?**

Use the worksheet on page 160 and the tips that follow as a guide when making a decision about whether to repair or upgrade your old equipment or purchase a new system.

- If the monitor indicator light is not coming on at all and you have checked all of the connections, you may have a bad monitor. In this case it may be cheaper to buy a new monitor. If you are considering a larger monitor or a flat screen, shop around. Both large monitors and flat screens have become more affordable.

- If the monitor indicator light is on but there is no picture, there is a good chance it could be the video card. A new video card is usually a reasonably priced option to consider.

- If the mouse is not working, the first thing to do is be sure the mouse driver is installed correctly.

- If the keyboard is not working, one way to troubleshoot is to try it on another computer. If it still doesn't work, a new keyboard is the practical solution. If it is a specialized keyboard, call the vendor to troubleshoot.

- If nothing happens when the computer is started, but the monitor light is on, there may be a problem with the CPU (the big box). If you take it to be fixed, ask the vendor to call you before they perform any repairs. If the repair is costly, you may want to consider buying a new unit.

- If you need a larger processor, you may want to call the vendor from whom you purchased the computer to see if it can be upgraded. If it is upgradeable, compare the price of an upgrade to a new unit.

- If memory is the problem, call the vendor to get an estimate on the cost of adding memory as well as how much memory can be added. Adding memory can be a cost-effective solution.

160

—

Computer
Resources
for People
with
Disabilities

Worksheet 9C: Repair vs. New Purchase

Problem	Cost to fix	Cost to purchase new
Monitor	_____	_____
Mouse or similar device	_____	_____
Keyboard or keyboard alternative	_____	_____
Hard drive	_____	_____
Larger processor	_____	_____
CD-ROM, DVD	_____	_____
Memory	_____	_____
AT, such as screen reader, Braille embosser, etc.	_____	_____

If you decide it would be a better investment to purchase a new device, consider all of your options. Ask yourself the following questions:

- What new technologies are available that may better fit my needs now and in the future?

- Is there a technology center nearby (or a upcoming technology conference) where I can see or try some of the new devices and software available?

- Is there an assistive-technology lending library in my state where I could try several devices, peripherals, and software before purchasing them to be sure they fit my needs?

- What new options would I like my computer to have?

    - Larger monitor

    - Flat screen

    - Drive that reads and writes CDs and/or DVDs

    - Other options

Last Thoughts

Whether you are a student, working, or retired, prepare to replace or upgrade your computer every three years. As new software is released and old software is upgraded, a faster processor, more memory, a larger hard drive, or a larger video card may be required. Your adapted peripherals and equipment may outlast some of these changes.

Keeping your computer and software up-to-date is an ongoing process. Be sure to budget for the necessary repairs and upgrades. Your relationships with vendors and a strong local support system will contribute to well-maintained equipment. Although none of us can foresee what changes the next few years will bring, you can be sure that the computers of the future will be able to do things we can't even imagine today.

Part II

The Technology Toolbox

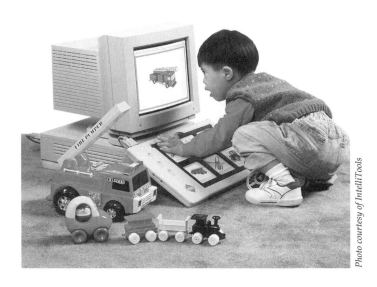

Contents

Using the Technology Toolbox

Many people start their search for technology by asking questions, and their questions often follow a similar pattern. The Technology Toolbox was created with knowledge of the most common questions, and it can help you develop your own route for navigating the technology solutions you will find. Rather than approaching the subject from the perspective of specific problems or disabilities, the Technology Toolbox approaches it from the viewpoint of the significant task to be done and a person's ability to perform that task. This approach reflects our philosophy that it is not the person with the disability who has the problem, but rather the environment that is deficient for failing to appropriately accommodate the individual's needs.

The Technology Toolbox was designed to provide you with information and ideas so you can be a good consumer of technology and make well-informed decisions. We provide information but do not suggest that any one approach or tool is right for you. Only you can make that determination.

How to Use the "Ask Yourself" Charts

Starting on page 169, you will find a set of charts that prompt you to ask yourself questions such as "How effectively can I see the computer screen?" or "How effectively can I use the keyboard?" To use the charts, start by finding the question that most closely fits the key issue that you, your child, your student, or your client faces as a potential limitation to using technology. If you have a number of issues to address, you will probably choose to employ more than one chart.

Next, in the far-left column of the appropriate chart, locate the ability level that most aptly describes your situation. In the second column, identify the difficulty or difficulties you feel you might encounter in attempting to use computer technology. (When there are multiple choices in a column, each is keyed to a symbol (● ■ ▲ ◆ ☆ ○). Then, in the third and fourth columns, locate the possible solutions and the tools to explore that are marked with the same symbols. In other words, for difficulties marked with ●, read the possible solutions marked with ● and the tools marked with ●. For difficulties marked with ■, read the possible solutions marked with ■ and the tools marked with ■. And so on.

Once you identify a tool that bears further investigation, turn to the product description for that item to learn more (page numbers are in parentheses).

How to Use the Product Descriptions

The product descriptions are intended to provide you with enough information to get a good feeling for the product without going into complex technical details. For each product you will get a sense of the range of available features and an understanding of why there may be a wide variation in cost—for example, because of differences in sound quality, speed, capacity, or user flexibility and friendliness.

Each product description lists related products that may also be useful. For more comprehensive information about specific assistive-technology products, the following resources will be helpful (see Part III for phone numbers and addresses):

Closing the Gap **Annual Resource Directory**.

Adaptive Device Locator System (ADLS), a database on CD-ROM containing the full range of adaptive- and assistive-technology products. This product is available from **Academic Software, Inc.**; Internet users can browse its contents at www.adaptworld.com.

CO-NET, a CD-ROM containing the Cooperative Electronic Library on Disability. This CD, available from the **Trace R&D Center,** contains several databases on assistive-technology products and vendors, service providers, and publications. It also contains copies of legislation and other relevant documents.

ABLEDATA, a database containing information on the full range of assistive-technology products. This database is included on the Trace CO-NET CD. You can also call the Trace R&D Center at (608) 263-1156, and a staff member will search the database for specific information for you. Additionally, you can contact the **National Rehabilitation Information Center (NARIC)** at (800) 346-2742.

Alliance for Technology Access Assistive Technology Hub, found at ataccess.org.

All the products in the Technology Toolbox meet the following criteria:

- They have been used successfully by people with disabilities.

- The manufacturer or the vendor generally offers customer support.

- They run on either a Macintosh or a PC (any exceptions are noted).

The inclusion of a product is not an endorsement of its suitability for any individual or situation. It is simply one product to consider in your search for solutions.

168

Computer
Resources
for People
with
Disabilities

It is true that specific information on technology is often out-of-date before it is printed—an inevitability in a field that is changing so rapidly. Companies expand, reduce, and merge, often changing addresses, phone numbers, and sometimes even names. Although we can't include tomorrow's products, we have listed today's key vendors. Part III includes an alphabetical listing of all the vendors mentioned in the Technology Toolbox, along with the most current information about them. Stay in touch with them; they offer new products on a regular basis. In addition, more and more people around the country are specializing in keeping track of what is happening in the AT field. Find and befriend them. Happy exploring!

Ask Yourself...How Effectively Can I See the Computer Screen?

★ My Abilities	Difficulties I Might Encounter	Possible Solutions	Tools to Explore
I see the screen well	● Small text ▲ Small cursor ■ Screen glare	● Increase text size ▲ Increase cursor size ■ Reduce glare	● Software features: easy-to-read screens (176) ▲ Software features: modified cursors (179) ■ Monitor additions (248)
I see the screen close up	● Monitor not close enough ■ Small monitor	● Modify position of monitor ■ Use large monitor ▲ Magnify screen	● ▲ Monitor additions (248) ■ Monitors ▲ Screen magnification software (245)
I see large text and graphics	Small text and graphics	● Magnify screen ■ Large-print program ☆ Use speech output	● Screen magnification software (245) ● Monitor additions (248) ■ Software features: easy-to-read screens (176) ☆ ■ Talking and large-print word processors (233) ☆ Screen readers (243) ☆ Speech synthesizers (240)
I use senses other than vision	Information is visual	◆ Use speech output ● Tactile output	◆ Screen readers (243) ◆ Speech synthesizers (240) ● Refreshable Braille displays (238) ● Braille embossers and translators (235)

TECHNOLOGY TOOLBOX

Ask Yourself…How Effectively Can I Use the Keyboard?

★ My Abilities	🔒 Difficulties I Might Encounter	🔑 Possible Solutions	🔧 Tools to Explore
I use two hands	● Task is tiring ■ Typing goes slowly ☆ Keys too close together ▲ Keys too far apart	◆ Use physical supports ● Accelerate input ■ Isolate keys ☆ Use small or programmable keyboard ▲	◆ Arm and wrist supports (216) ● Word prediction programs (223) ■ ▲ Alternate keyboards (181) ● ■ Macro programs and abbreviation expansion programs (220) ● Voice recognition systems (200) ☆ Keyboard additions (190)
I use one hand	◆ ● Must hit two keys at a time ▲ Typing goes slowly ○ Keys too close together	◆ Latching keys ● ▲ Alternate keyboard layouts ■ Accelerate input ○ Isolate keys	◆ Access utilities (187) ▲ ■ Alternate keyboards (181) ■ Macro programs and abbreviation expansion programs (220) ■ Word prediction programs (223) ■ Voice recognition systems (200) ○ Keyboard additions (190)
I point	● ■ ☆ Limited use of hands ▲ Keys too close together ○ Typing goes slowly	● Larger keys ■ Point and type ○ Accelerate input ☆ Use on-screen keyboard with mouse alternative ▲ Isolate keys	○ ● Alternate keyboards (181) ☆ Trackballs (214) ■ Pointing and typing aids (208) ○ Voice recognition systems (200) ☆ Touch screens (210) ○ Macro programs and abbreviation expansion programs (220) ☆ Electronic pointing devices (206) ○ Word prediction programs (223) ▲ Keyboard additions (190)
I use one or more controllable movements	Physically accessing keyboard	◆ Use speech input ● Use switch input	◆ Voice recognition systems (200) ● Switches and switch software (193) ● Interface devices (196)

Ask Yourself...How Effectively Can I Use the Mouse?

★ My Abilities	🔒 Difficulties I Might Encounter	🔑 Possible Solutions	⚒ Tools to Explore
I can make hand movements	Relating the mouse to the screen	● Use direct selection ▲ Use mouse replacements	● ▲ Touch screens (210) ▲ Joysticks (212) ▲ Alternate keyboards (181)
I can make *some* hand movements	◆ Fine motor dexterity ■ Gross motor dexterity	◆ Use gross movements ■ Use fine movements	◆ Alternate keyboards (181) ■ Trackballs (214) ■ Joysticks (212) ■ Access utilities (187)
I can use other controllable movements	Manipulating mouse	☆ Use mouse replacements	☆ Pointing and typing aids (208) ☆ Electronic pointing devices (206) ☆ Switches and switch software (193) ☆ Interface devices (196) ☆ Joysticks (212)

TECHNOLOGY TOOLBOX

Ask Yourself...How Effectively Can I Interact with Information?

★ My Abilities	🔒 Difficulties I Might Encounter	🔑 Possible Solutions	🔧 Tools to Explore
I can interact with auditory support	Written instructions, directions, or prompts	● Use programs with verbal instructions, directions, and prompts	● Speech synthesizers (240) ● Software features: auditory cues (178) ● Talking and large-print word processors (233)
I can interact with written support	Verbal instructions, directions, or prompts	◆ Use programs with written instructions, directions, and prompts	◆ Software features: visual cues (178) ◆ Operating system
I understand information	▲ Maintaining attention ■ Inaccessible format	● Use motivating and interesting approaches ▲ Simplify methods of input ■ Create accessible format	▲ ● Talking and large-print word processors (233) ● Speech synthesizers (240) ▲ Joysticks (212) ▲ Touch screens (210) ▲ Software features: easy-to-read screens, instructional choices (176, 177) ▲ Alternate keyboards (181) ■ Optical character recognition, scanners (203)
I can interact with limited information	Excessive or overwhelming information	◆ Limit information presented ● Use graphics ■ Provide fewer keys	◆ Software features: instructional choices (177) ● Software features: graphics (177) ■ ● Alternate keyboards (181)
I can interact with some of the environment	Understanding cause and effect	▲ Train in cause/effect skills	▲ Switches and switch software (193) ▲ Touch screens (210) ▲ Alternate keyboards (181)

Ask Yourself... *How Effectively Can I Read (Comprehend)?*

★ My Abilities	🔒 Difficulties I Might Encounter	🔑🔒 Possible Solutions	🔧 Tools to Explore
I read at a lower than expected level	Reading at expected level	● Have computer speak text ■ Isolate text into manageable chunks ☆ Transfer print materials to computer ◆ Train in reading comprehension	● Speech synthesizers (240) ● Talking and large-print word processors (233) ■ Software features: easy-to-read screens (176) ☆ Optical character recognition and scanners (203) ◆ Reading comprehension programs (224)
I comprehend single sentences	Too many words at a time	● Have computer speak text ■ Isolate text into manageable chunks ☆ Transfer print materials to computer ▲ Train in reading comprehension ◆ Support reading with graphics	● Speech synthesizers (240) ● Talking and large-print word processors (233) ■ Software features: easy-to-read screens (176) ☆ Optical character recognition and scanners (203) ▲ Reading comprehension programs (224) ◆ Software features: graphics (177)
I comprehend single words	Decoding	■ Practice letter recognition ☆ Practice letter-sound recognition	■ Reading comprehension programs (224) ☆ Alternate keyboards (181) ☆ Speech synthesizers (240)
I comprehend the meaning of symbols	Understanding words	◆ Use graphic symbols ● Have computer speak text	◆ Reading comprehension programs (224) ◆ Software features: graphics (177) ◆ Alternate keyboards (181) ◆ Speech synthesizers (240) ◆ Talking and large-print word processors (233) ● Software features: auditory cues (178)

Ask Yourself...How Effectively Can I Write (Compose)?

★ My Abilities	🔒 Difficulties I Might Encounter	🗝️ Possible Solutions	🔧 Tools to Explore
I write at a lower than expected level	◆ Organizational skills ■ Writing ideas	■ Train in composition	◆ ■ Writing-composition programs (228)
I can compose single sentences	◆ Vocabulary ● Grammar/syntax ▲ Spelling ■ Writing ideas	◆ Support vocabulary ● Support grammar ▲ Support spelling ■ Train in composition	◆ Electronic reference tools (230) ● ▲ Word prediction programs (223) ◆ ▲ Software features: built-in utilities (179) ● ■ Writing-composition programs (228)
I can combine words and phrases	Communicating meaning	● Train in composition ■ Enter whole words and phrases	● Writing-composition programs (228) ■ Alternate keyboards (181)
I need to use alternatives to writing	Communicating meaning	◆ Use graphics with voice output ● Speak sentences to computer	◆ Software features: custom programs, graphics (180, 177) ◆ Alternate keyboards (181) ◆ Speech synthesizers (240) ● Voice recognition systems (200)

My Abilities	Difficulties I Might Encounter	Possible Solutions	Tools to Explore
I understand how to handle equipment	● ◆ Physical manipulation ▲ ■ ○ Reading print materials and manuals	● Create access to disks ■ Create access to system ◆ Create access to printer ▲ Request accessible format ○ Create accessible format	● Hard disk drives ■ Electronic aids to daily living (258) ◆ Printers ○ Braille embossers, translators (235) ▲ Software features: clear documentation (177) ○ Screen readers (243) ○ Speech synthesizers (240) ○ Reading machines (263) ○ Optical character recognition and scanners (203)
I can physically handle equipment	Comprehending task	◆ Simplify entry to programs and files ● Simplify disk operation	◆ Operating system ● Hard disk drives

TECHNOLOGY TOOLBOX

Software Features

The following features, available as options in many operating systems and some software programs, may be helpful to someone who needs support to access a computer. You may want to keep these features in mind when you explore and compare software.

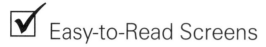 Easy-to-Read Screens

Screens that are easy to read and understand can make a critical difference for many users. Features to consider include the following:

- clear, uncluttered screens, which may reduce distraction

- simple and legible text

- menu items that are represented with both graphics and text, with options for large characters

- ability to alter the style, font, or spacing of text

If voice software will be used, programs that place text in one column, rather than in multiple columns, can be read more easily. Multiple columns or boxes of text are very difficult for screen reading software to interpret. Similarly, asterisks or other nonalphabetical characters used for decoration can make it more difficult to use a screen reader. For example, the user might hear "asterisk, asterisk, asterisk" or "dash, dash, dash."

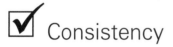 Consistency

Consistent placement of menus and objects on the screen or on a series of similar screens makes using a program more intuitive and predictable. A consistent layout provides easier navigation for users of screen magnification software, because they know where to look for things. It may also assist users with mobility disabilities by minimizing the need to move the mouse unnecessarily. Consistency supports the use of software that employs "markers," which identify fixed locations on the screen where particular menus or objects are found. These locations are "marked," and the cursor jumps to the mark when a switch or key is pressed.

Also important for consistency are objects, menus, and content that respond uniformly throughout the program, present clear options as needed, and clarify the consequences of making choices.

Logical Labels

Programs generally present the user with a series of choices, either in a list or on a menu. These choices should be labeled with logical, understandable names that give the user a reasonable sense of what will happen when a specific choice is made. This is particularly important when the user—such as someone using a screen reading program—is dependent on auditory cues.

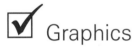 # Instructional Choices

Instructional software programs generally allow parents or teachers to control content and lesson presentation. The difficulty level, vocabulary, sound, timing, speed, and amount of graphics and text presented can often be adjusted.

Some programs of this type keep track of the student's record or progress. Some also allow parents or teachers to personalize content by adding customized spelling lists, vocabulary lists, or math problems.

Graphics

Graphics can be used to encourage interaction or to convey information in interesting and motivating ways. Graphics or icons may be used as alternatives to words or commands, providing access to nonreaders. Some programs use cues that involve color (for example, "find the red sock"). Other programs allow you to import or scan in graphics—such as a picture of your dog—to add personal content.

Graphics can play a role in supporting reading. Graphics without text, however, may limit access to those with visual disabilities, including individuals with color blindness.

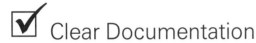 # Clear Documentation

Easy-to-understand software manuals, whether provided by the software developer or by a third party, can be important. Many include easy-to-follow diagrams and illustrations of what should be on the screen. Some manuals are available in large print, in Braille, on audiocassette, on computer disk, or in a print layout that is easy to use with a scanner or reading machine.

SOFTWARE FEATURES

178

Computer
Resources
for People
with
Disabilities

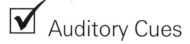# On-Screen Instructions

Some programs provide on-screen instructions—in the form of help lines, help balloons, or help windows—and instructional prompts to guide the user through the program. It is best if the user has control over how long these instructions remain on the screen.

Auditory Cues

The form of prompts and instructions—verbal, written, or animated—is often critical to making a program accessible and, for some people, easier to understand. Some programs are written to offer verbal prompts or instructions that use synthetic (computer-generated) speech and might require a speech synthesizer. Others use digitized (recorded) speech, sounds, or music and might require a sound card. At times, both sound and visual indicators are used simultaneously and are noticeable even when one's full attention is not on the screen. Some programs use auditory prompts or signals to get the user's attention, which can be helpful for some users (whose attention may wander quickly from the computer program) but distracting for others. If the user needs full auditory access to the program, make sure the program provides enough auditory prompts to be useful. Some programs include limited auditory functions designed to enhance the program for a sighted user, and these functions may not cover enough aspects of the program to make it a reasonable alternative for a nonsighted user.

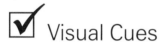# Visual Cues

Some programs use visual prompts at different times during program operation to assist the user in understanding the task. When visual cues accompany auditory cues, more complete access to the program is provided. This can be important to people who do not benefit from auditory cues.

An example of visual cueing is prompted writing, which is a feature that allows a facilitator to guide the writer in creating sentences or stories by providing step-by-step written instructions that appear in a box on the screen. These directions usually don't print out as part of the written assignment and are invisible to the person who reads the final product.

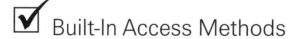# Built-In Access Methods

Some programs have built-in alternative access methods and allow you to select the option you want. You can choose to have the program accept input from alternative devices—such as a single switch, alternate keyboard, joystick, touch screen, or game controller—in lieu of the standard keyboard and mouse. Some programs change the presentation of the program to match the requirements of the device. For example, if "single switch" is selected, the program might change from a point-and-click selection method to one that scans the available choices.

 # Built-In Utilities

Many conventional software programs, such as word processors, spreadsheets, and databases, come with utilities as part of their package. These utilities may include spell checkers, visual "zoom" options, dictionaries that allow for modifications, a thesaurus, macros, abbreviation expansion capabilities, and grammar checkers. Some programs also come with text-to-speech options in their menus. Having these utilities built into the software program eliminates the need to run multiple programs simultaneously. This helps to reduce system conflicts and makes it easier to navigate between features.

 # Alternatives to a Mouse

Some operating-system utilities and software packages allow the user to use keyboard commands in place of a mouse, which is helpful for individuals who find it difficult or impossible to use a mouse. This is accomplished by using the arrow (or cursor) keys or by pressing a specific combination of keys (keyboard equivalents) that activate the desired function. Be aware that some programs provide a way to operate only certain parts of the program by keyboard and require a mouse to do the rest.

 # Modified Cursors

A cursor is the pointer or marker—typically a small flashing square, two crosshairs, an I-beam, or an arrow—that indicates where you are on the screen. Cursors come in a variety of forms. Many computer operating systems and a number of software programs allow the user to select from a range of cursor options. The options might include a larger arrow, a thicker I-beam, a hand, a pointed finger, a pencil, thick crosshairs, an animated figure, or even a snake!

180

Computer
Resources
for People
with
Disabilities

✓ Creation of Custom Programs

Authoring programs—for example, HyperStudio (Knowledge Adventures), Authorware, and Director (Macromedia)—allow users to build their own tutorials, drill and practice software, communication boards, instructional aids, informational resources, animations, and other styles of software. A wide range of users—from students to business professionals—can create programs of their own using authoring software. Most authoring programs allow you to work with graphics, text, sounds, and video. The more customized and sophisticated you want your program to be, the more knowledge you will need of the program language and tools.

Custom authoring programs are also available for several assistive or augmentative communication devices, such as Overlay Maker (IntelliTools), Speaking Dynamically (Mayer-Johnson), and Talking Screen (Words+, Inc.).

Alternate Keyboards

Alternate keyboards offer a variety of ways to provide input to a computer through keyboards that vary in size, layout, and complexity. Some available varieties of alternate keyboards are described below.

Programmable keyboards are versatile and often can be programmed so that letters, numbers, words, or phrases can be entered by pressing customized keys. They can be larger in size than a standard keyboard, allowing for a

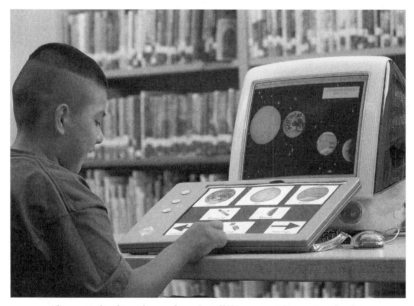

Alternate keyboards, such as IntelliKeys, can be customized to match the needs of any software program.
(Photo courtesy of IntelliTools)

larger target area. Smaller keys can also be set up so less range of motion is required. Overlays are used to define the customized keyboard layout.

Miniature keyboards are designed with keys spaced close together to allow someone with a small range of motion or only one hand to access all the keys. They are typically lightweight and small in size.

182

Computer
Resources
for People
with
Disabilities

Chording keyboards generally have a limited number of keys. Text is entered by pressing combinations of keys. The keys are sometimes programmable so that certain combinations will enter custom words or phrases.

On-screen keyboards are images of a standard or modified keyboard placed on the computer screen by software. The keys are selected by using a mouse, touch screen, trackball, joystick, switch, or electronic pointing device.

 Use this tool to...

Simplify the method of entering information

Create keyboards using pictures instead of words or letters

Create keyboards using tactile materials to represent words or letters

Type with words and phrases instead of letters

Access communication boards

Communicate your meaning through graphics, photographs, or objects

Practice letter-sound recognition

Learn the meaning of words through graphics, photographs, or objects

Limit the number of keys to the specific ones required to do the task

Enter information using a switch with an on-screen keyboard

Replace the mouse

Enter information by head movement or eye gaze with an electronic pointing device and an on-screen keyboard

Enter information using a mouse or mouse alternative with an on-screen keyboard

Provide easy-to-use, motivating activities

 Potential users...

Interact with limited information and benefit from structured choices

Use two hands, but find the task tiring

Use two hands, but find the keys too far apart

Use one hand, but type slowly

Combine words and phrases (rather than letters) to communicate meaning

Use alternative methods of writing, through symbols and speech

Have limited fine motor skills

Can point, but need an alternative when the task is designed for full use of hands

Need to operate a computer without the use of hands

Comprehend single words, but require help with decoding

Communicate through language-based symbols or graphics

Comprehend the meaning of graphic symbols rather than letters

Have limited gross motor skills

Have visual impairments that limit the ability to discriminate keys

See keys that have higher visual contrast

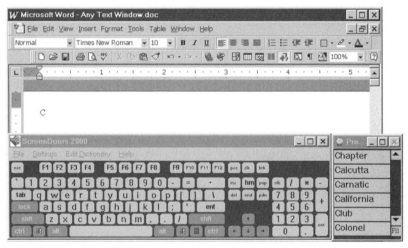

ScreenDoors 2000 replaces your physical keyboard with one that is on-screen. (Photo courtesy of Madentec)

 ## Features to consider

Some can be customized for different key sizes and arrangements

Some need software that translates the keyboard functions to the computer

Some have an internal computer interface; others require an external one

Some allow the standard keyboard and the alternate keyboard to be used at the same time

Some require less pressure to activate a key

Some on-screen keyboards come with dictionaries or word/letter-prediction programs

184

Computer
Resources
for People
with
Disabilities

Some replace the mouse and keyboard

Some replace the keyboard only

Some can customize the color contrast between the keys and the background

Some can be used to create a series of keyboard layouts by making overlays

 Cost

Programmable keyboards

Range: $150–900   Common: $150–500

Miniature keyboards

Range: $80–800   Common: $80–200

Chording keyboards

Range: $200–650   Common: $300

On-screen keyboards

Range: $0–800 (this product may be built into or bundled with another product at no additional cost.)

Common: $200–500

 Common vendors

Programmable keyboards

EKEG Electronics Company, Ltd.

Exceptional Computing, Inc.

Fentek Industries, Inc.

Hatch Associates

Handykey Corporation

Inclusive TLC

IntelliTools, Inc.

Keyboard Alternatives & Vision Solutions, Inc.

Madentec Limited

TASH International, Inc.

Zygo Industries, Inc.

Miniature keyboards

EKEG Electronics Company

In Touch Systems

Keyboard Alternatives & Vision Solutions, Inc.

TASH International, Inc.

Chording keyboards

AccuCorp, Inc.

Bellaire Electronics

Handykey Corporation

Infogrip, Inc.

Keyboard Alternatives & Vision Solutions, Inc.

Keybowl, Inc.

On-screen keyboards

Applied Human Factors

Crick Software

Gus Communications

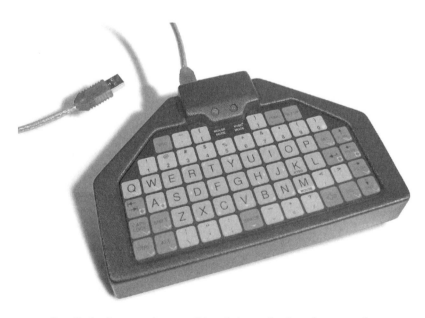

Small-size keys, such as on this miniature keyboard, ensure that
a small range of motion allows full access to the keyboard.
(Photo courtesy of TASH International, Inc.)

186

———

Computer
Resources
for People
with
Disabilities

Inference Group: Dasher Project

Innovation Management Group, Inc.

IntelliTools, Inc.

Lake Software

Madentec, Ltd.

Mayer-Johnson Company

Microsoft Corporation

Prentke Romich Company

R. J. Cooper and Associates

Words+, Inc.

 Additional information

The layout and key size of the standard keyboard is not always the best choice for access. Alternate keyboards provide different means of accessing a computer. Some alternate keyboards can be modified and the layouts customized for individual use. Paper or plastic overlays fit on top of the keyboard and are used to designate where to press on the keyboard for a desired keystroke or customized response. The areas to be pressed can be defined by letters, numbers, punctuation, words, pictures, tactile materials, or objects. Many innovative teaching strategies can be implemented using an alternate keyboard.

Chording keyboards often come with a tutorial for learning chord combinations and a quick reference chart of chord combinations. The hand size the device accommodates may be limited (for example, some are sized for an adult, male hand only). The number of keys varies among devices (12 finger keys and six thumb keys, 10 finger and four thumb, etc.). Software may allow for a reconfiguration of the chords. Additional software utilities—such as abbreviation expansion programs—can be used with a chording keyboard to increase typing speed by reducing keystrokes. Braille note takers are another chording device.

On-screen keyboards may have built-in scanning options to be used with a single switch.

 Related products

Arm and wrist supports

Electronic pointing devices

Joysticks

Keyboard additions

Pointing and typing aids

Speech synthesizers

Switches and switch software

Talking and large-print word processors

Touch screens

Trackballs

Access Utilities

Access utilities are software programs that modify various aspects of the standard keyboard to simplify operation of the keyboard, replace the mouse, substitute visual cues for sound signals, or add sound cues to keystrokes.

 Use this tool to...

Increase speed when using a pointing aid or typing device

Change the layout of the keyboard

Limit the entering of unwanted keys

Provide other indicators (visual or auditory) when some key functions are on or off

Eliminate the need to press more than one key at a time

Enhance visibility of system cursors for pointing and editing

Provide auditory feedback regarding keys pressed and screen elements (icons, etc.) being accessed

 Potential users...

Use one finger or a pointing aid and need to increase speed or reduce the number of keystrokes required

Have better gross motor dexterity than fine motor dexterity

Use only one hand, but the task requires pressing two keys at a time

Strike keys by mistake because of tremors

Require visual notification of computer alert sounds

Require auditory feedback to access the user interface

Use alternate input devices

188

Computer
Resources
for People
with
Disabilities

 Features to consider

Some allow access to menus through function keys or combinations of keystrokes

Some eliminate the need to press two keys at a time

Some can adjust the key repeat rate

Some can adjust the time required to hold a key down before it is entered

Some prevent the keyboard from accepting two quick presses of the same key (repeat defeat)

Some let the user replace the mouse and use the number pad on the keyboard to control cursor movements

Some indicate if keys such as Num Lock, Scroll Lock, and Caps Lock are on or off

Some replace computer sounds with visual indicators

Some allow the user to redefine the keyboard to create other layouts

Some allow the user to replace the computer keyboard with a virtual one

Some allow the user to access the user interface through auditory feedback

 Cost

Range: $0–1,200 (This product may be built into or bundled with another product at no additional cost.)

Common: $150

 Common Vendors

Apple Computer, Inc.

Baum Retec AG

Gus Communications

IBM Independence Series Information Center

IntelliTools, Inc.

The Matias Corporation

Microsoft Corporation

Microsystems Software, Inc.

R. J. Cooper and Associates

Silicon Graphics, Inc. (SGI)

Words+, Inc.

 Additional Information

Macintosh: The system software for Macintosh computers comes with two "Universal Access" control panels—called Easy Access and CloseView—that have many customization features. They offer a variety of keyboard and output adjustments, depending on the version of the system software that you are using. Check your Macintosh user's manual for more information. Depending on the source of the computer, these control panels are not always preinstalled but are included in a Universal Access folder on the system installation CD. In the Macintosh OS X operating system, these features are included in the Universal Access Preferences. These new access tools offer almost complete keyboard access to the Macintosh computer for the first time. In Mac OS X 10.2 and later, even more access features are included, such as built-in text-to-speech and magnification. More information about these and other access features can be found at Apple's website (www.apple.com/macosx/jaguar/universalaccess.html).

PCs: All versions of Windows since Windows 95 offer a number of accessibility options that are built into the software itself. For more information about these features and about which version of Windows supports a particular access feature, you can visit the "Accessibility Support" page at Microsoft's website (www.microsoft.com/enable). In Windows 98, the user can install the Accessibility Options program, which includes the Accessibility Wizard and the Magnifier. The Accessibility Wizard customizes options for vision, hearing, and mobility. The Magnifier displays an enlarged section of the screen in a separate window. Windows 2000 and Windows XP add a Narrator for limited text-to-speech and an on-screen keyboard.

AccessX, a standard set of utilities similar to the Accessibility Options built into Microsoft Windows or Mac OS X, can be installed on all of the variants of Unix (like Linux and FreeBSD). These operating systems also offer a growing number of other options for accessibility. Best of all, these tools are all free; however, they require more patience in configuring and installing than their other, more established counterparts in Windows and MacOS. More information on these tools can be found on the Trace website (http://trace.wisc.edu/linux/).

190

Computer
Resources
for People
with
Disabilities

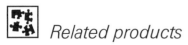 *Related products*

Abbreviation expansion and macro programs

Joysticks

Keyboard additions

Pointing and typing aids

Trackballs

Word prediction programs

Keyboard Additions

A variety of accessories have been designed to make keyboards more accessible. They include the following:

Keyguards — hard plastic covers with holes for each key. By using a keyguard, someone with an unsteady finger or with a pointing device can avoid striking unwanted keys.

Moisture guards — thin sheets of plastic that protect keyboards from spills and drooling.

Alternative labels add visual clarity or tactile information to the keys.

 Use this tool to...

Keyguards

Increase accuracy

Maintain correct placement of hand while typing

Moisture guards

Protect from spills and other moisture

Alternative labels

Provide cues for frequently used keys

Increase color contrast on the tops of the keys

Provide Braille cues

Assist new typists in learning the keyboard

Provide cues for spelling or finding letters

Potential users...

Need more separation between the keys to accommodate a mouthstick, pointer, or assistive typing device

Need more separation between the keys

Benefit from visual or tactile enhancement of the keyboard

Benefit from guarding keys from accidental pressing

 Features to consider

Keyguards must match the specific keyboard layout

Moisture guards must match the specific keyboard layout

Some labels add color to specific keys

Some labels add tactile cues to the keys

Some labels enlarge the name or include the function of specific keys

 Cost

Keyguards

Range: $50–200   Common: $100

Moisture guards

Range: $12.95–55   Common: $35

Alternative labels

Range: $0–20 (This product may be built into or bundled with another product at no additional cost.)

Common: $10

 Common vendors

Keyguards

Assistech

IntelliTools, Inc. (for Intellikeys)

Keytools, Ltd.

Maxess Products, Ltd.

Prentke Romich Company

192

Computer
Resources
for People
with
Disabilities

TechAble

Turning Point

Words+, Inc.

Moisture guards

Don Johnston, Inc.

Enabling Devices

Hooleon Corporation

Turning Point

Alternative labels

Ai Squared

Carolyn's Products for Enhanced Living

Data Cal Corporation

Don Johnston, Inc.

Enabling Devices

Hooleon Corporation

Inclusive TLC

 Additional information

Keyguards are available for many of the alternate keyboards. Many stationery stores carry printed labels that can be put on keys to enlarge letters and numbers or to increase the color contrast. Note: small stickers (such as press-on earrings) that can be used to highlight important keys may be purchased at a "dollar" store.

 Related products

Access utilities

Alternate keyboards

Arm and wrist supports

Braille adaptations

Monitor additions

Pointing and typing aids

Talking and large-print word processors

Switches and Switch Software

Switches offer ways to provide input to a computer when a more direct access method, such as a standard keyboard or mouse, is not possible. Switches come in various sizes, shapes, colors, methods of activation, and placement options. An interface device and software are usually required to connect the switch to the computer and to interpret the operation of the switch.

Some software programs have been developed specifically for use with a switch and can employ on-screen scanning. With on-screen scanning, the computer highlights (either by sound, visual cue, or both) options available to a user about what action he or she wants the computer to take. Using these specialized products, when a visual or auditory prompt indicates a desired keyboard or mouse function, the user activates the switch and the desired function occurs.

Other programs have built-in options to allow switch use. Many standard software programs can be accessed through a switch with the use of additional software and devices.

 Use this tool to....

Enter text or data when using the keyboard is not feasible

Interact with the computer by selecting choices as they are highlighted

Set up a series of responses using multiple switches

Train in cause and effect

Facilitate choice making

Control the computer via Morse code

 Potential users...

Need an alternative to the keyboard

Need to operate a computer with only one or two movements

Benefit from structured interaction with the environment

 Features to consider

Most can be mounted and activated by any part of the body

Some are activated by pressure (the pressure required may vary from switch to switch)

194

Computer
Resources
for People
with
Disabilities

Some are sensitive to light touch

Some are activated by sound

Some are activated by interrupting a light beam

Some can be fastened to any part of the body

Some are activated by pulling

Some are activated by squeezing

Some are activated when bent

Some are available in different sizes and colors

Some are activated by the blink of an eye

Some are activated by a specific motion detected by a digital camera

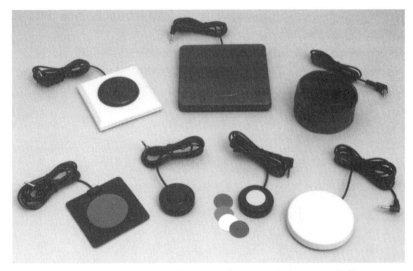

*Single switches come in a wide range of sizes and shapes and allow you
to do anything on the computer that anyone else can do.
(Photo courtesy of TASH International, Inc.)*

 Cost

Range: $0–400 (This product may be built into or bundled with another
product at no additional cost.)

Common: $40–65

 Common vendors

Switches

Ability Research, Inc.

AbleNet, Inc.

Adaptivation

Don Johnston, Inc.

Edmark Corporation

Enabling Devices and Toys for Special Children

Exceptional Computing, Inc.

GenesisOne Technologies, Inc.

Hatch Associates

KY Enterprises/Custom Computer Solutions

Luminaud, Inc.

ORCCA Technology

Prentke Romich Company

TASH International, Inc.

Zygo Industries, Inc.

Switch software

Academic Software, Inc.

Assistive Technology, Inc.

Computers to Help People, Inc.

Consultants for Communication Technology

Don Johnston, Inc.

Easter Seals Colorado

Edmark Corporation

Gus Communications

IntelliTools, Inc.

Laureate Learning Systems, Inc.

Madentec, Ltd.

MarbleSoft

Mayer-Johnson Company

NanoPac, Inc.

Prentke Romich Company

R. J. Cooper and Associates

Simtech Publications

196

Computer
Resources
for People
with
Disabilities

Soft Touch/KidTech

Switch In Time

UCLA Intervention Program for Young Handicapped Children (UCLA/LAUSD)

Visuaide 2000, Inc.

Words+, Inc.

 Additional information

Switches can operate everything from environmental controls, augmentative and alternative communication devices, and appliances to battery-operated toys and radios. They can also control powered mobility. A switch and switch interface will operate programs designed for single-switch or dual-switch input. Some programs that require a single input (mouse click, space bar, return key, etc.) may also work with a switch interface. For access to the entire keyboard and most commercial programs, additional software and hardware are required.

Switches can be home-made or custom-made by rehabilitation practitioners or at rehabilitation facilities.

 Related products

Interface devices

Joysticks

Interface Devices

Interface devices provide access to the standard alphanumeric keyboard, the keyboard functions, and sometimes the mouse controls by enabling the use of single switches, alternate keyboards, or other input devices.

Switch interfaces are used to connect the switch to the computer and are used with software written for single-switch use.

Multiple-switch interfaces are used to connect a series of switches to the computer. Each switch can be defined as a character, word, phrase, or action.

Multiple-input interfaces are used to connect switches, alternate keyboards, and other input devices to the computer. Software that interprets the information from these devices for the computer is often included. These devices can allow the user to operate software with a switch even when the software wasn't originally written for switch use.

When switches are used, the choices of letters, numbers, or pictures are displayed and sequentially highlighted on the screen. When the highlight indicates the desired choice, the user activates the switch, which enters the choice into the computer. This selection process is called *scanning*.

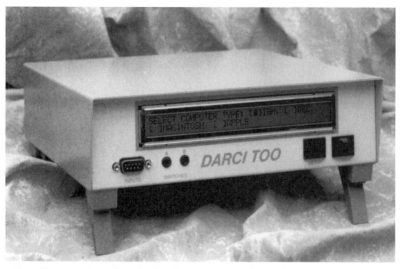

Darci Too, an interface device, lets you control a wide range of computers using switches, joysticks, video-game controllers, and expanded keyboards. (Photo courtesy of WesTest Engineering Corporation)

 Use this tool to...

Enter text or data when using the keyboard is not feasible

Design customized keyboards to simplify activities

Make communication boards that can be accessed by a switch or alternate keyboard

Set up a series of responses or keyboard functions, one for each switch, using multiple switches

Enter text by sending Morse code through one or two switches

Use standard software programs through a switch-scanning method

Connect a switch, and use software with built-in scanning options

 Potential users...

Need to operate a computer without the use of their hands

Use switches, alternate keyboards, or directional joysticks to operate a computer

198

Computer
Resources
for People
with
Disabilities

Need to operate a computer with only one or two movements

Have difficulty with direct selection and/or isolating a finger-point

 Features to consider

Most include the ability to control the rate at which the selections are highlighted when scanning is used

Some keyboard interfaces operate with any software program

Most can work while the standard keyboard and mouse remain active

Some can use pictures or graphics, instead of text, to indicate choices

Some show the highlighted choices on the computer screen

Some show the highlighted choices through a built-in display on the interface device

Some can replace the mouse

Some allow a variety of methods for selecting the choice (for example, the choice is made when the switch is pressed versus when it is released)

Some can interpret Morse code

Some can work with a speech synthesizer for auditory prompts to indicate choices

Some have built-in word prediction capabilities

 Cost

Switch interfaces

Range: $75–500   Common: $100

Multiple-switch interfaces

Range: $75–275   Common: $100

Multiple-input interfaces

Range: $400–1,000   Common: $500–800

 Common vendors

Switch interfaces

AbleNet, Inc.

Consultants for Communication Technology

Crick

Don Johnston, Inc.

Gus Communications

Hatch Associates, Inc.

IntelliTools, Inc.

R. J. Cooper and Associates

TASH International, Inc.

Multiple-switch interfaces

AbleNet, Inc.

Crick

Don Johnston, Inc.

IntelliTools, Inc.

R. J. Cooper and Associates

TASH International, Inc.

Multiple-input interfaces

AbleNet, Inc.

Don Johnston, Inc.

IntelliTools, Inc.

R. J. Cooper and Associates

TASH International, Inc.

WesTest Engineering Corporation

Words+, Inc.

 Additional information

Some software programs have built-in scanning. All that is needed is a simple switch interface to connect the switch to the computer.

Some standard software programs can be operated by a switch. This requires an interface device that connects the switch to the computer and includes software that creates the choices and interprets the switch activation.

Morse code can be used to enter text into the computer by using switches. One, two, or three switches may be used, depending on the needs of the user. Doing this requires an interface device that connects the switch to the computer and includes software that interprets the code.

200

———

Computer
Resources
for People
with
Disabilities

PC/Windows users must carefully select software for the on-screen display to make sure it is compatible with other programs and with the operating system, especially when using Windows. Hardware solutions offer the advantage of being independent of software compatibility problems, but may require the user to visually attend both to the computer screen and to a separate scanning device.

 Related products

Abbreviation expansion and macro programs

Alternate keyboards

Joysticks

Speech synthesizers

Switches and switch software

Word prediction programs

Voice Recognition Systems

Different types of voice recognition systems—also called *speech recognition systems*—are available. Voice recognition allows the user to speak to the computer instead of using a keyboard or mouse to input data or control computer functions. Voice recognition systems can be used to create text documents such as letters or e-mail, to browse the Internet, and to navigate among applications and menus by voice. In the past, two different types of voice recognition software were available—continuous speech and discrete speech. With the advances in computing power that have taken place in both PCs and Macs, continuous-speech software is the only version widely available today.

 Use this tool to...

Input text or data by voice

Navigate among files, applications, and menus by voice

Execute standard commands by voice

Control all functions of a computer hands-free

 Potential users...

Have difficulty using a standard keyboard and mouse due to motor-skills issues or repetitive-stress injuries

Have learning disabilities resulting in some difficulties with spelling or grammar

Use dictation (instead of a keyboard) as their method of typing

 ## *Features to consider*

Most systems must be trained to respond to a particular voice (the user reads a predetermined list of words or a passage into the computer microphone to provide the user's unique information on pronunciation and inflection)

Most systems require the user's speech to be consistent

Discrete dictation systems require the user to pause slightly between words and are generally more forgiving of differences in speech or articulation

Continuous dictation systems use more fluent and natural speech patterns and are more successful with users who have good enunciation and who use organized and sequenced speech

Many allow the user to navigate the computer—that is, to control the cursor and execute commands—by voice

Some have larger vocabularies and provide a wider range of navigation or dictation capabilities

Some include vocabularies specific to a vocational field (e.g., legal, medical)

Some dictation systems can recognize phrases that the user uses frequently

Some can recognize a wide range of voices and do not require training

Some computers have voice navigation built into their system

 ## *Cost*

Range: $50–700 Common: $150

 ## *Common vendors*

Apple Computer, Inc.

Commodio

ScanSoft

IBM Corporation

Microsoft Corporation

202

Computer
Resources
for People
with
Disabilities

 Additional information

Discrete vs. continuous speech: Initially, all speech recognition programs required discrete speech, meaning at least a short pause between words. This made the analysis of the sounds and determination of the word spoken an easier computing task. It also made the system somewhat more forgiving of speech differences. Almost all systems are now moving toward a more natural, continuous-speech model. It is more intuitive, especially for new users, and is made possible by more powerful processors and more sophisticated recognition models. Experience to date has shown that continuous-speech software is becoming more tolerant of speech differences; users with mild to moderate speech impairments have successfully trained continuous-speech recognition programs. Additionally, many of the hands-free command and control options available in the discrete-speech products are now being incorporated into most continuous-speech recognition products.

Readiness: A user's readiness for use of voice recognition includes such factors as understanding the operating system and software to be used, being able to sustain attention, and coping with frustration during the training process.

Environmental factors: Consider the environment in which the system will be used, such as at home, at work, or in a classroom. Background noise can affect the system, which generally needs to be used in an environment consistent with the one in which the training was done. Confidentiality issues must also be addressed, as all input is spoken aloud.

Support and training: Thorough training in the use of the software is very important for success with voice recognition. Some users may require customized training and equipment along with high levels of support. Post-training support is also a key issue. Technical difficulties often arise with the voice recognition software, application software, operating system, or hardware. Proper computer setup and troubleshooting can be especially critical if voice recognition is the main computer input method for an individual with a disability.

Hardware: All hardware is not created equal. A compatible combination of software, microphone, sound card, and computer are required for successful voice recognition. The software should be chosen first and then tried on the intended computer before a final purchase is made. This is especially true if you work on a laptop.

Macintosh: Apple Plain Talk, a program for dictation and navigation, is an extension of System 7.1 and later versions. To do dictation, you need a product that will enable both dictation and navigation. In the newest versions of Mac OS X (10.2 and up), Apple has included an updated speech recognition program that takes the place of Plain Talk; it is called Apple Speech and is found under the Speech Preferences. IBM has a version of its ViaVoice software available for the Macintosh.

PC: Windows requires a program specifically designed to allow navigation in its environment. Most voice recognition products require an appropriate sound card—specifically a multichannel card, such as the SoundBlaster Live! or TurtleBeach Montego Bay cards. Most Windows voice applications are continuous-speech models, and the most popular are those by ScanSoft (formerly made by Dragon Systems). For users of the Open Source Operating Systems, such as Linux or FreeBSD, IBM offers a version of its ViaVoice software. There are also some free products being developed, but none are at a user-friendly stage of development at this time.

 Related products

Electronic aids to daily living

Optical character recognition software and scanners

Optical Character Recognition Software and Scanners

Optical character recognition (OCR) software works with a scanner to convert print from a printed document into a standard computer text file.

A scanner is a device that converts an image from a printed page to a computer file. With OCR software, the image of the print is converted to computer text that can then be edited. Pictures and photographs do not require OCR software because OCR software is only for text, not graphics. Scanners usually come with OCR software and graphics-scanning software included.

 Use this tool to...

Transfer a printed worksheet to the computer so it can be accessed by assistive devices

Convert printed documents into computer text so they can be read aloud by a speech synthesizer, printed in large text, or embossed in Braille

Transfer printed materials to the computer to change text size, style, and layout

204

———

Computer
Resources
for People
with
Disabilities

 Potential users...

Can handle the equipment physically but cannot read printed manuals
or documents

May be unable to see the printed text in materials or documents

Are teachers or parents preparing accessible materials for a child with a
disability

May write with adaptive computer devices

May read at a lower level than their potential

Need materials in an accessible format to complete an activity

 Features to consider

All OCR programs translate text from print form into a computer text
file, which can then be edited

Most OCR programs adjust for scanning single or multiple pages

Some scanners have a document feeder for multiple-page documents

Most OCR programs have light adjustment

Many OCR programs automatically detect and adjust for page
orientation (portrait or landscape)

Some OCR programs can be set to scan a whole page or selected portions
of a page

All scanners have utility programs that allow the scanner to
communicate with the computer and save the scanned image as a
graphic file on the computer

Most scanners are capable of detecting colors

All handheld scanners can scan small portions of text at one time

All flatbed scanners can scan full-size pieces of paper at one time

Some scanners require the installation of an interface board in order to
communicate with the computer

 Cost

OCR programs

Range: $0–1,200 (This product may be built into or bundled with another
product, such as a scanner, at no additional cost.)

Common: $600

Scanners

Range: $50–3,000   Common: $150

 Common vendors

OCR software

ABBYY USA

CAD & Graphics

Freedom Scientific, Inc.

Kurzweil Educational Systems Group

Scanners

Epson

Hewlett-Packard Company

Microtek

UMAX Technologies, Inc.

Visioneer

Additional information

OCR software is invaluable in converting materials from print to electronic formats. The OCR software translates the print into computer text by comparing the scanned-in materials against a table of letters, numbers, and symbols, and makes a best guess as to what each character represents. The resulting file can then be altered like any other computer text file.

Scanners come in two varieties: flatbed and handheld. Flatbed scanners look very much like desktop copiers. Handheld scanners are held in the hand. Flatbed scanners are great for scanning full-sized images and multiple pages at high resolutions (the amount of detail that a scanner can perceive), but cost substantially more than the handheld variety.

People with hand/arm motor issues may have difficulty using handheld scanners.

Scanners, with their accompanying software, are available for use on both Macintosh and PC platforms. Most scanner software does not distinguish between pictures and text. To the scanner, everything is just an image. To obtain computer text that can be edited, OCR software is needed. Copyright laws must be respected when scanning printed material.

206

Computer
Resources
for People
with
Disabilities

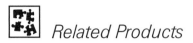 *Related Products*

Reading machines

Screen readers

Electronic Pointing Devices

Electronic pointing devices allow the user to control the cursor on the screen using ultrasound, an infrared beam, eye movements, nerve signals, or brain waves. When used with an on-screen keyboard, electronic pointing devices also allow the user to enter text or data.

 Use this tool to...

Enter text or data into a computer when a mouse and/or keyboard are not feasible

Operate a draw program or a computer-aided design program

Actuate an on-screen keyboard

Operate assistive communication systems and environmental controls

Access the Internet

 Potential users...

Need to operate a computer without the use of their hands

Have good head control, eye control, or the ability to learn control through nerve signals or brain waves

 Features to consider

Some require activating a switch to make a selection

Some allow the user to pause or dwell on a key to select it

Some require an eye blink to make a selection

All work with an on-screen keyboard

Some allow the user to control the cursor by head motions

Some require the head to be held still while the computer is controlled with eye movements

Some have wires connecting them to the computer; others operate remotely

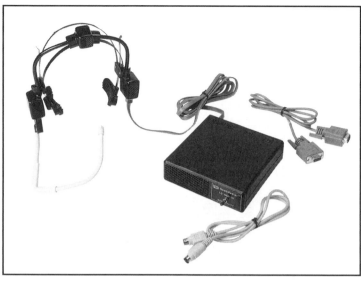

*The HeadMaster provides full mouse control for people who are
unable to use their hands but have good head control.
(Photo courtesy of Prentke Romich Company)*

 ## Cost

Range: $200–6,500   Common: $1,500

 ## Common vendors

Boost Technology

Brain Actuated Technologies

Eye Control Technologies, Inc. (dba NaturalPoint)

EyeTech Digital Systems

Madentec, Ltd.

Origin Instruments Corporation

Prentke Romich Company

Technos America, Ltd.

Words+, Inc.

 ## Additional information

Once the cursor has been placed in the desired location, the user can make a
selection by dwelling on a particular location or by using one of a variety of
switches. The pointer will work with any on-screen keyboard compatible

208

Computer
Resources
for People
with
Disabilities

with the computer system. Electronic pointing devices that rely on eye movements or nerve impulses are newly emerging and are rapidly becoming more sophisticated and economically viable.

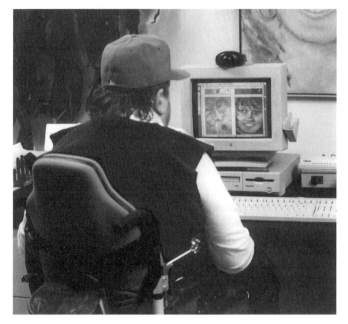

Bill Miller shows how Tracker can be used to help him in his career as a graphic designer. (Photo courtesy of Madentec)

 Related products

Alternate keyboards

Switches and switch software

Word prediction programs

Pointing and Typing Aids

A pointing or typing aid is typically a wand or stick used to strike keys on a keyboard. They are most commonly worn on the head, held in the mouth, strapped to the chin, or held in the hand.

 Use this tool to...

Enter text or data using a standard or alternate keyboard

Operate a trackball, touch screen, or alternate keyboard

Potential users...

Need to operate a computer without the use of their hands

Need to point with a single digit or an extension of a digit

 Features to consider

All can be used with keyguards

All can be used with standard, alternate, or modified keyboards

Most are adjustable in length and fit

Many can be used with switches or augmentative communication devices to turn pages or perform daily living activities

Some have an adjustable head strap to be worn on the head or across the chin

Some have a bite plate to be held in the mouth

Some are used with a splint on the hand or arm

 Cost

Range: $15–600   Common: $130

 Common vendors

Extensions for Independence

Independent Living Aids, Inc.

North Coast Medical, Inc.

Sammons Preston Rolyan—An AbilityOne Company

 Related products

Access utilities

Alternate keyboards

Touch screens

Trackballs

Touch Screens

A touch screen is a device placed on the computer monitor (or built into it) that allows direct selection or activation of the computer by a touch of the screen.

 Use this tool to...

Provide an intuitive interface for young children and those with cognitive disabilities

Build cause-and-effect skills

Encourage computer use

Enter text or data using an on-screen keyboard

Make a direct selection by pointing at the screen instead of using the mouse

 Potential users...

Need a more intuitive interface

Need a more direct method of moving the cursor on the screen

Need a simpler method of input

Require interesting and motivating approaches

Need a clear connection between their actions and the computer's reactions

 Features to consider

All allow direct selection of items on the screen by touching a monitor

All take the place of the mouse

Some are integrated into the monitor

Some are detachable from the monitor

Some require software specifically written to work with the touch screen

Most can be used with an on-screen keyboard

Most are available in several sizes to accommodate different-sized monitors

Cost

Range: $200–5,000   Common: $350–2,000

 Common vendors

Edmark Corporation

KEYTEC, Inc.

3M Touch Systems

Troll Touch

 Additional information

Touch-sensitive screens may be used to move a cursor, imitate a mouse, or make selections. The touch screen may be used as one large single switch with some switch software. Some users point and type on an on-screen keyboard using a touch screen to provide a direct cognitive connection between the keys and the screen. The mouse and keyboard may still be used while the touch screen is active.

When the software includes simple point-and-click options, touch screens are effective with young children or people whose skills are at a lower functional level. Touch screens tend to be most effective when used with programs where the target or active area is as large as the individual's fingertip. A stylus, with a soft point, can be used for greater accuracy.

A consideration in the purchase of a touch screen is the continued lifting of the arm to activate the window. Raising the arm could prove tiring over time for some individuals. On the other hand, the same motions could be incorporated into the individual's therapy to improve gross motor skills.

Macintosh: The detachable screen plugs into the Apple Desktop Bus (ADB) port or the Universal Serial Bus (USB) port on the back of the computer. It functions transparently as a mouse replacement with all software programs.

PCs: The detachable screen plugs into the serial port or the Universal Serial Bus (USB) port on the back of the computer. Other types of screens may be built directly into the monitor. Most versions for PCs require special drivers (utility programs) that are supplied with the touch screen. The screen will only work with programs that involve the use of a mouse.

212

Computer
Resources
for People
with
Disabilities

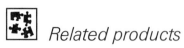 *Related products*

Alternate keyboards

Pointing and typing aids

Speech synthesizers

Switches and switch software

Joysticks

A joystick may be used as an alternate input device. Joysticks that can be plugged into the computer's mouse port can control the cursor on the screen. Other joysticks plug into game ports and depend on software that is designed to accept joystick control. Four types of control are offered by joysticks: digital, optical, glide, and direct. Digital control allows movement in a limited number of directions, such as up, down, left, and right. Glide, optical, and direct controls allow movements in all directions (360 degrees). Direct-control joysticks have the added ability to respond to the distance and speed with which the user moves the stick.

 Use this tool to...

Encourage computer use

Operate a communication system or environmental-control unit

Activate the computer with different parts of the body

Enter text or data using an on-screen keyboard

Practice mobility skills for operating a power wheelchair

Play a game

 Potential users...

Have use of their hands, but encounter problems when the task requires relating the mouse movement to the screen

Need to operate a computer without the use of their hands

Interact well with information but need a simpler method of input

Interact well with information but require interesting and motivating approaches

Practice use of a joystick for wheelchair control

Features to consider

Some specially designed joysticks allow access to popular game-stations

Some are equipped with up to three control buttons that can be programmed to perform various functions or accept alternate switches

Some require more force to operate than others; alternatively, the force can be adjusted

Some are designed to be operated with the chin or head

Some work only with software written specifically for use with joysticks

Some offer switch adaptation

Some are wireless

 Cost

Range: $14–500   Common: $50

 Common vendors

Compusult Limited

Fellowes

Gravis

KY Enterprises

Logitech

Penny and Giles Computer Products, Ltd.

Prentke Romich Company

R. J. Cooper and Associates

TASH International, Inc.

 Additional information

Joysticks come in many sizes and shapes. Available options include the capacity for audio feedback, mounting hardware, and cables allowing use with different computers. Some interface devices accept joysticks as an input method. There are literally hundreds of companies that manufacture or distribute joysticks. Those listed above are just a few.

Macintosh: Joysticks can plug directly into the mouse or USB port and control the cursor on the computer screen in all programs.

214

Computer
Resources
for People
with
Disabilities

PCs: The joystick may plug into the mouse, serial, or USB port and may need software for mouse emulation.

 Related products

Interface devices

On-screen keyboards

Switches and switch software

Trackballs

Trackballs

A trackball looks like an upside-down mouse, with a movable ball on top of a stationary base. The ball can be rotated with a pointing device, a hand, or another body part.

 Use this tool to...

Enter text or data with an on-screen keyboard

Perform mouse functions using fewer hand movements or a pointing aid

 Potential users...

Have fine motor skills but lack gross motor skills

Use a pointing aid to manipulate the cursor

Control a single finger well

Need to separate the cursor-position function from the clicking function

 Features to consider

Some have buttons that lock in the down position for easy dragging

Some have buttons that are programmable to perform computer operations

Some have adjustable cursor speed and sensitivity

Some are designed for maximum comfort of the user and may be adjusted for left- or right-hand use

Some have balls available in a variety of diameters, ranging from one inch to four inches

Some allow for switches to be connected and used as a mouse function

Many have keyguards available as an accessory

Many are now cordless, which adds flexibility to the placement of the trackball

 Cost

Range: $25–170   Common: $75–130

 Common vendors

Cirque Corporation

Ergo Kare, Inc.

Fellowes

Kensington Microware, Ltd.

Keytools, Ltd.

Logitech, Inc.

Microsoft Corporation

Penny and Giles Computer Products, Ltd.

 Additional information

A trackball is a mouse alternative used to control cursor movements and actions on a computer screen. The cursor is activated when buttons on the device are pressed, similar to the operation of a standard mouse. Some have features that allow you to click and drag with a single finger or pointer. Make sure there are no compatibility issues when adding a trackball or joystick.

A variety of companies sell trackballs. Check discount stores for the best prices!

 Related products

Alternate keyboards

Joysticks

Touch screens

Arm and Wrist Supports

Arm supports are devices that stabilize and support the arms and wrists while the user is typing, using a mouse or trackball, or performing other tasks. Wrist rests support the wrist while it is resting but should not be used when striking the keys.

 Use this tool to...

Maximize comfort and reduce risk of injury when typing or using a cursor control device.

 Potential users...

Need support to avoid fatigue or pain

Benefit from having their arms stabilized

 Features to consider

Most provide support at the arm or wrist

Some attach to the table in front of the computer

Some include cuffs to support the forearm

Some offer adjustable heights

Some swivel in two or more directions

Some mount on the chair instead of the table

Some wrist supports are built into the keyboard

 Cost

Arm supports

Range: $87–600   Common: $100

Wrist supports

Range: $10–20   Common: $15

Common vendors

AliMed, Inc.

DS Ergonomics

Ergo Kare, Inc.

Keyboard Alternatives and Visions Solutions, Inc.

Saunders Ergo Source

XYBIX Systems

 Additional information

One or both arms can be supported in a variety of ways, depending on individual preference. Before the release of commercial products, people used foam wedges, foam bars, and other types of support.

 Related products

Alternate keyboards

Keyboard additions

Monitor additions

Product Descriptions: Processing Aids

Browsers and Browser Add-Ons

The *Internet* is the term used to describe the multitude of large and small computers around the world that are linked by cables, modems, telephone lines, and satellites. Many individuals, organizations, and companies use the Internet to offer websites with information or opinions in the form of text, graphics, and—increasingly—sounds and video.

To access these websites you must have a browser on your computer. Browsers are software programs that interpret the code used to create websites and present it in an intelligible format.

Standard browsers usually come with a new computer or may be downloaded from the Internet for free. These browsers may have some access features already built in. For some of these browsers, add-ons are available to enhance accessibility. Some browsers assume the user has accessibility needs and provide speech output and other advanced aids. Finally, several general accessibility programs—particularly screen readers—may include custom commands to assist with Internet access.

Like all other computer programs, browsers pose considerations for users with disabilities in that your methods of providing input and perceiving output must be addressed in order to use them.

Even with browsers maximized for accessibility, it is important to realize that the accessibility of specific websites is primarily determined by the conscientiousness of the people who designed them. For example, some screen readers and other speech-output programs can read ALT tags, which are text descriptions associated with pictures. However, for this to work properly, the page's programmer has to add the ALT tag to the page and make sure it provides useful information (e.g., it is not helpful to label a photo with the ALT tag "photo"). If you are interested in finding out more about creating accessible websites, an excellent resource is WebAIM (www.webaim.org).

 Use this tool to...

"Surf" or browse the millions of websites and resources on the Internet

Locate information of potential interest to you using various "search engines"

Keep a record of sites you have visited during current and past Internet sessions

Download files to your computer, including software, utilities, graphics, or text files

Shop for or order items of interest to you

 Potential users…

Need or want quick access to news, information, and opinions on a variety of topics

Need or want access to information and reference material in alternative formats

Need or want to conduct their shopping, banking, socializing, etc., from home

 Features to consider

Most work best on computers with faster processors and connection speeds

Most allow the user to set text size, color, and fonts for viewing web pages

Most have options to turn graphics, sounds, or video on or off

Most allow the user to choose which website comes up each time the browser is opened

Some have built-in text-to-speech support

 Cost

Browsers

Range: $0–40   Common: free

Accessible Browsers and Browser Add-Ons

Range: $0–1,000   Common: $250

 Common Vendors

Standard Browsers

America Online

Lynx

220

Computer
Resources
for People
with
Disabilities

Microsoft Corporation

Mozilla

Netscape Communications

Opera Software

Accessible Browsers and Browser Add-Ons

AbleLink Technologies

Code-It Software, Inc.

Eco-Net International

Freedom Scientific, Inc.

IBM Accessibility Center

ION Systems

J. Bliss

Qwerks.com, Inc.

Serotek Corporation

Texthelp Systems Ltd.

 Additional Information

See Internet Resources in Part III for more information.

 Related products

Abbreviation expansion and macro programs

Alternate keyboards

Electronic pointing devices

Screen magnification software

Screen readers

Word prediction programs

Macro Programs and Abbreviation Expansion Programs

Macro programs allow a user to "record" a long series of commands and assign them to a function key, a combination of keys, a menu item, or an on-screen button. Once a macro is recorded, the user can execute the complicated task exactly as recorded simply by typing the assigned key(s), selecting from the menu, or clicking the button. For example, with one or two keys you could open a word processor, enlarge the text, and enter your name or address. You might create another macro to save and print your document in one keystroke.

Abbreviation expansion programs allow the user to assign a series of letters, words, or sentences to one or more keystrokes. When the assigned keys (the abbreviations) are entered, the program will automatically insert the expanded text. Abbreviation expansion is sometimes used to speed vocabulary selection with an augmentative communication system.

 Use this tool to...

Assign simple keystrokes to frequently used words, phrases, sentences, or paragraphs

Automate a series of events, such as locating a word processor, starting it up, setting the text to a large size, entering the date at the top, and setting the margins

Create a simple communication tool by storing phrases that can be entered by a keystroke into a word processor and read aloud by a speech synthesizer

Store phrases that can be entered by a switch interface, an alternate keyboard, or a communication device

 Potential users...

Benefit from using fewer keystrokes

Need to increase speed

Need to perform repetitive tasks on the computer accurately and efficiently

Need shortcuts or reminders for difficult tasks

 Features to consider

Many can be used with the operating system as well as with most software programs

Some can be found as a feature of other programs, such as word processors and word prediction programs

Some come with pre-stored abbreviations for specific fields of study

Some can record mouse movements

222

Computer
Resources
for People
with
Disabilities

Some can use multiple characters as the abbreviation

Some can use only single characters as the abbreviation

Some require two or more keys to be typed simultaneously

Some allow the user to create on-screen buttons for each macro

Some can open Internet browsers and go to particular websites

 ## Cost

Range: $20–500   Common: $80–150

 ## Common vendors

Active Words Systems, Inc.

Apple Computer, Inc.

CE Software, Inc.

Corel, Inc.

Gus Communications

IBM Corporation

Microsoft Corporation

TASH International, Inc.

Words+, Inc.

 ## Additional information

Many abbreviation expansion features are combined with word prediction programs. Many word processors and standard office software come with built-in macro features. Many of the standard software companies have built macros into their software, as well as the ability to design customized macros.

 ## Related products

Access utilities

Word prediction programs

Word Prediction Programs

Word prediction programs enable the user to select a desired word from an on-screen list located in the prediction window. This list, generated by the computer, predicts words from the first one or two letters typed by the user. The word may then be selected from the list and inserted into the text by typing a number, clicking the mouse, or scanning with a switch.

 Use this tool to...

Increase written productivity and accuracy

Increase vocabulary skill through word prompting

Reduce fatigue by eliminating unnecessary keystrokes

 Potential users...

Can recall the first few letters of a word but need assistance with spelling to produce written work

Benefit from word prompts to build vocabulary skills

Need to increase speed or reduce keystrokes

Need assistance with word recall

 Features to consider

All have prediction windows that appear on the screen

Most can be used with common word processing programs

Some allow users to add their own words

Some can customize text size and the position of the word list on the screen

Some can present word choices alphabetically or by frequency of use

Some predict words based on rules of grammar

Some make predictions based on the user's pattern of word usage

Some automatically capitalize the first word in a sentence

Some provide built-in scanning features that visually or auditorily highlight word choices

Some can use text-to-speech programs to speak the selection or the completed sentence

Some are packaged with abbreviation and expansion features

224

Computer
Resources
for People
with
Disabilities

 Cost

Range: $100–1,000   Common: $300–500

 Common vendors

Applied Human Factors

Aurora Systems, Inc.

Don Johnston, Inc.

Gus Communications

Madentec, Ltd.

Prentke Romich Company

Texthelp Systems Ltd.

Words+, Inc.

 Related products

Abbreviation expansion and macro programs

Access utilities

Reading Comprehension Programs

Reading comprehension programs focus on establishing or improving critical thinking, vocabulary, and reading skills through ready-made activities, stories, exercises, or games.

 Use this tool to...

Improve reading level and comprehension skills

Practice letter-sound recognition

Increase understanding of words by adding graphics, sound, or animation

Develop decoding skills

Provide letter-sequence practice for word building

Provide word-sequence practice for sentence building

Improve word recognition

Increase vocabulary

Potential users...

Read at a level lower than their potential

Comprehend single sentences

Comprehend single words

Comprehend the meaning of symbols

 Features to consider

Some allow adjustment of the vocabulary level

Some offer speech output

Some have placement tests

Some do student record keeping

Some have supplementary materials for use off of the computer

Many provide graphics

Some provide animation and sound

Some highlight text as it is read aloud

Some allow adjustment of the font size

Some allow the user to record written or spoken notes

Some provide icons on menu bars or in menus

Some speak items in menus or dialog boxes

Some include built-in scanning for switches

 Cost

Range: $25–2,000   Common: $50–100

 Common vendors

Center for Applied Special Technology (CAST), Inc.

Compass Learning, Inc.

Compu-Teach

Creative Learning Company

Discis Knowledge Research, Inc.

Don Johnston, Inc.

Educational Activities, Inc.

226

Computer
Resources
for People
with
Disabilities

Freedom Scientific, Inc.

Great Wave Software

Houghton Mifflin School Division

IBM Independence Series Information Center

K–12 MicroMedia Publishing

Knowledge Adventure

Kurzweil Educational Systems Group

Laureate Learning Systems, Inc.

The Learning Company

Lexia Learning System, Inc.

Little Planet Software/A Division of Houghton Mifflin

MarbleSoft

MECC (see Riverdeep)

Millenium Software

Milliken Publishing Company

Mindplay

Optimum Resources, Inc.

Riverdeep & Edmark Corporation

Scholastic Software

Siboney Learning Group

Sunburst Communications/A Division of Houghton Mifflin

SVE and Churchill Media

Taylor Associates Communications

Tom Snyder Productions

William K. Bradford Publishing Company

 Additional information

The software may start at the level of letter recognition and move sequentially to the level of passage comprehension, or it may focus only on a more limited set of reading comprehension skills.

Most reading comprehension programs now come in CD-ROM versions, which allow for greater voice output, graphics, and animation. The size of the text, the complexity of the graphics and text on the screen, and the level of voice output vary greatly from program to program.

Related products

Optical character recognition and scanners

Speech synthesizers

Talking and large-print word processors

Reading Tools and Learning-Disabilities Programs

Reading tools include software designed to make text-based materials more accessible for people who struggle with reading or reading materials. Options may include scanning, reformatting, navigating, or speaking text aloud.

 Use this tool to…

Change the size, style, and spacing of written text for people with low vision

Hear printed text spoken aloud

Create easy-to-navigate "electronic books" from printed or electronic text

Add or modify graphics

 Potential users…

Read at a level below their potential

Comprehend better when they simultaneously hear and see text highlighted

Have difficulty seeing or manipulating conventional print materials

Have emerging literacy skills or are learning English as a second language

 Features to consider

Some allow scanning and viewing of the original page

Some allow adjustment of the font style, size, and spacing as needed

Some highlight text as it is spoken

228

Computer
Resources
for People
with
Disabilities

Some allow insertion of written or spoken notes

Some provide a button bar with icons for reading or navigation

Some have built-in switch scanning for reading or navigating the text

 Cost

Range: $200–2,000   Common: $400

 Common vendors

Freedom Scientific Learning Systems Group

CAST, Inc.

Kurzweil Educational Systems Group

 Additional information

These tools vary greatly in price as well as in features offered, such as acquisition of text, options for reading, and user customization. As with all assistive technologies, the user is encouraged to try the various options before purchasing the software to make sure the tools provided meet their individual needs.

 Related products

Optical character recognition and scanners

Reading comprehension programs

Screen readers

Talking and large-print word processors

Writing-Composition Programs

Writing-composition programs provide a structured environment that enhances an individual's ability to produce written material.

 Use this tool to...

Teach brainstorming, concept mapping, creative writing, journal writing, and classification

Develop outlines and main ideas, write first drafts, and learn how to proofread

Learn sentence completion, story completion, and proper sequencing

Facilitate communication using graphics and speech output

 Potential users...

Are reluctant writers

Write at a level lower than their potential

Compose simple single sentences but require writing ideas and prompts

Combine words and phrases but need help to communicate meaning and organize content

Use an alternative to traditional writing methods

 Features to consider

Most offer activities at various levels to develop writing skills

Some provide teacher/parent materials to allow for individualization based on the user's needs

Some include prewriting activities

Many include writing-development activities

Some provide graphics to use in place of written words

Some offer choices for how material is presented

Many provide voice output

Some include text prompts on-screen to use as guides

Some include graphics combined with text

Some offer visual organization displays

 Cost

Range: $30–325   Common: $100

 Common vendors

Communication Skill Builders

Crick Software

Don Johnston, Inc.

230

Computer
Resources
for People
with
Disabilities

Humanities Software

Inspiration Software

IntelliTools, Inc.

Knowledge Adventures

Mayer-Johnson, Inc.

Microsoft Corporation

Riverdeep/The Learning Company

Scholastic Software

Slater Software

Sunburst Communications/A Division of Houghton Mifflin

Teacher Support Software

Tom Snyder Productions

 Additional information

There are a vast number of writing-composition programs available for both Macintosh and PC computers that make it possible to match programs to individual user needs at different skill levels. Most of these products are standard educational programs.

 Related products

Abbreviation expansion and macro programs

Electronic reference tools

Software features: Built-in utilities

Talking and large-print word processors

Electronic Reference Tools

Electronic reference tools provide the user with ways to access traditional print materials and resources via the computer. Such references include dictionaries, thesauruses, atlases, almanacs, encyclopedias, and professional journals.

Use this tool to...

Access traditionally print-based materials via computer

Transfer information, definitions, images, or statistics into a word processing program

Electronically search for a specific name, date, word, or topic

Complete academic course work

Interact with multisensory reference materials

 Potential users...

Need access to reference materials in formats other than print

Interact well with information but require interesting and motivating approaches

Need clear, direct access to information

 Features to consider

Many are available on CD-ROM disks and hold huge volumes of information

Some are available free or for a subscription rate through the Internet

Some are accompanied by photos, music, sounds, video clips, animation timelines, or tables

Most allow a variety of search options

Most provide some standard computer operations, such as copy, paste, and print

Some are available in languages other than English

 Cost

Range: $0–2,000 (Sometimes new computers include reference software as part of their standard software package)

Common: $100

 Common vendors

Franklin Electronic Publishers, Inc.

Freedom Scientific Learning Systems Group

232

Computer
Resources
for People
with
Disabilities

Houghton Mifflin

Microsoft Corporation

SVE and Churchill Media

WizCom Technologies, Ltd.

 Additional information

Some of the most widely used electronic reference tools found on the Internet are listed below:

www.diccionarios.com/index.phtml

www.library.northwestern.edu/reference/electronic_reference/

www.ldresources.com/resources/confusing_words_resources.html

www.m-w.com/

www.pdictionary.com/spanish/

http://dictionary.reference.com/

http://encarta.msn.com/

http://freedict.com/onldict/spa.html

 Related products

Built-in utilities

PDAs

Talking and Large-Print Word Processors

A talking word processor is software that provides auditory feedback as a person types text into the computer. The speech feedback is created through speech synthesis and can be set to speak each letter, each word, and/or each sentence depending on the needs of the individual using the software.

 Use this tool to...

Talking word processors

Have text spoken aloud by chosen parameters (letter, word, sentence, selected text)

Practice letter-name recognition

Combine graphics with speech

Provide a motivating and interesting element to the task

Provide confirmation of a keystroke without looking at the screen

Create a simple communication board using an alternate keyboard

Large-print word processors

View large-text options without losing full view of the program (the printed document will be normal in size and font)

 Potential users...

Need auditory feedback to help them focus their attention

Need auditory feedback to recognize letters, words, and/or sentences

Need auditory confirmation of the words they have typed

Potential users for Zoom features on software...

Need enlarged text, but do not want the final product to be enlarged when printed or sent to others

Need text specifically formatted to be readable

Need large text

234

Computer
Resources
for People
with
Disabilities

 Features to consider

All talking word processors speak the selected text aloud

Most talking word processors allow the option of hearing auditory feedback of letters, words, or sentences

Any combination of the preceding three is also possible as an option for feedback

Most talking word processors offer both speech feedback and text-enlarging options

Most talking word processors include speech-editing capabilities for correcting the pronunciation of a word

Some talking word processors have talking spell-check capabilities

Some talking word processors have word prediction capabilities

Some talking software can be used to enhance a regular word processor, thus turning it into a talking word processor

Most offer a variety of speech controls and options

Most talking word processors highlight the words and sentences as they read

Some talking word processors also offer the option of graphics to go with a word

 Cost

Range: $0–$1,700 (This product may be built into or bundled with another product at no additional cost.)

Common: $100

 Common vendors

Talking word processors

Center for Applied Special Technology (CAST)

Don Johnston, Inc.

IntelliTools, Inc.

Meyer Johnson, Inc.

Texthelp Systems Ltd.

Large-print word processors

Corel Software

Microsoft Corporation

 Additional information

A talking word processor does not generally have all the capabilities of a screen reader. While a few talking word processors provide screen reading outside of the word processing document, most do not.

Most word processing software can enlarge and change font in order to accommodate different size and print needs. Zoom is a feature built into Microsoft software and Word Perfect software. With Zoom, an individual can enlarge the print to whatever size is needed, on the monitor only. When the document is printed, the font will remain the normal size. Zoom is not like a screen magnification program. It only magnifies the letters within the text when they are on the screen.

 Related products

Screen readers

Braille Embossers and Translators

A Braille embosser translates computer-generated text into embossed Braille output on paper. Translation programs convert text produced on a computer by optical character recognition software working with a scanner or generated via standard word processing programs into formatted Braille that can be sent to an embosser.

 Use this tool to...

Emboss computer-generated Braille documents, including math, text, and graphics

Produce Braille materials, including books, handouts, signs, restaurant menus, and maps

 Potential users...

Are businesses, organizations, and educational institutions that need to produce accessible documents for the blind

Are students and adults who require Braille instead of standard print

236

Computer
Resources
for People
with
Disabilities

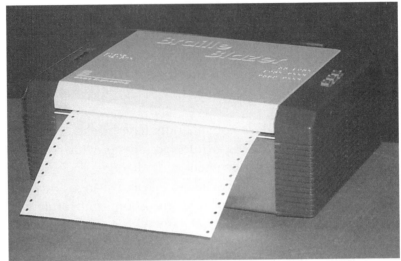

*A Braille printer such as Braille Blazer can print out text files in
Braille format. (Photo courtesy of FreedomScientific.com)*

 Features to consider

All emboss Braille

Most need translation software to create grade-two Braille, unless it is
produced by a Braillist on the computer using a Braille word processor

Some use speech to help users navigate through embosser options
menus

Some have liquid crystal displays to indicate page count

Some emboss graphics

Some emboss on two sides of a page (interpoint Braille) in one pass

Some produce both Braille and standard ink print on the same page

Some embossers may produce different sizes of Braille dots, such as
Jumbo Braille and eight-dot cell Braille, as well as the normal six-dot cell
or Braille character

Some embossers can be placed in a sound enclosure to reduce noise

 Cost

Embossers

Range: $1,700–40,000   Common: $3,000–4,500

Translators

Range: $200–1,000   Common: $595

 Common vendors

Embossers

American Thermoform Corporation

Beyond Sight, Inc.

Canadian National Institute for Braille

Enabling Technologies

Freedom Scientific, Inc.

Index Braille

ViewPlus Technologies

Translators

Duxbury Systems, Inc. (includes the former Braille Planet and Raised Dot Computing)

GW Micro

NFBTRANS (National Foundation for the Blind)

Optical Braille-recognition software

Neovision S.R.O.

Pulse Data/HumanWare, Inc.

 Additional information

Braille embossers are available in two categories: those designed for individual use and those designed for high-volume production of embossed materials. Some embossers can use serial, parallel, or wireless connections to a computer, and some can be networked.

If extreme accuracy in Braille translation and formatting is critical for the end user, a skilled Braillist must edit the Braille output of translation software since there are many exceptions and rules that currently cannot be incorporated into translation programs. In addition to software for translating computer text into Braille, software also exists that works with a scanner to translate Braille into text.

238

Computer
Resources
for People
with
Disabilities

 Related products

Note takers

PDAs

Reading machines

Refreshable Braille displays

Screen readers

Wireless

Refreshable Braille Displays

Refreshable Braille displays provide tactile output of information presented on the computer screen. Unlike conventional Braille, which is permanently embossed onto paper, refreshable Braille displays are mechanical in nature and lift small, rounded plastic or metal pins, as needed, to form Braille characters.

Refreshable Braille displays contain 18 to 80 Braille cells. After the line is read, the user can "refresh" the display to read the next line.

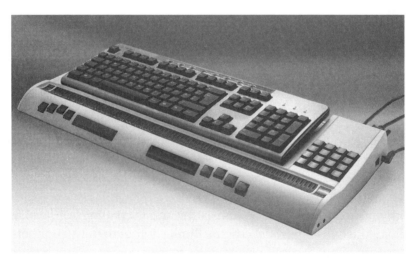

A refreshable Braille display provides tactile feedback from the computer for Braille users, including those with hearing impairments. (Photo courtesy of Pulse Data HumanWare, Inc.)

Use this tool to...

Display commands, prompts, and electronic text in Braille

Allow the user to get precise information about text attributes, screen formatting, and spelling on the computer display

Provide computer access to people who are visually impaired, where speech output might not be practical or desired

 Potential users...

Need to use Braille access to a computer

Prefer to use Braille access to a computer rather than speech

Prefer to use a combination of Braille and speech access to get the benefits of both

Need Braille for job tasks for which it is better suited than speech, such as precise text editing or working with programming code

 Features to consider

All can display text from the computer screen

Some can show an 80-column screen on a single Braille line

Some can indicate text attributes, such as upper case, highlighted text, and boldface

Some have a touch cursor, which enables the user to move the computer cursor to a particular character with the touch of a button located directly above it

Some have controls for reviewing screen contents, with the Braille display conveniently located on the front panel

Some function as part of a portable personal data assistant for people who are blind and can also be used on a computer as a refreshable Braille display

 Cost

Range: $3,500–15,000   Common: $4,500–8,000

 Common vendors

Alva

240

Computer
Resources
for People
with
Disabilities

Freedom Scientific, Inc.

Papenmeier

Pulse Data

 Additional information

No refreshable Braille access is currently available for Macintosh computers.

Some manufacturers of screen reading programs provide facilities for using refreshable Braille displays for screen access.

Some devices connect to a parallel port, while others connect to either a serial or a USB port on PCs.

 Related products

Braille embossers and translators

Note takers

PDAs

Screen readers

Speech Synthesizers

With appropriate software, a speech synthesizer can receive information going to the screen in the form of letters, numbers, and punctuation marks, and then "speak" it aloud.

 Use this tool to...

Hear computer text spoken aloud

Practice letter-sound recognition

Provide a motivating and interesting element to a task

Provide confirmation of a keystroke without looking at the screen

Hear auditory prompts and feedback from a screen reading program or talking word processor

Listen to text from manuals and documents transferred to the computer using an optical character recognition program and a scanner

Potential users...

Read at a level lower than their potential but benefit from text spoken aloud

Comprehend single words but require decoding skills

Comprehend the meaning of symbols but need to hear words

Require manuals and documents read aloud

Need auditory support when screen text is too small

Need auditory feedback to navigate the screen and select commands

Need materials in an accessible format to complete activities

Benefit from auditory feedback

Understand information but need to maintain attention on the task at hand

Use auditory feedback when information on the screen is unusable

 Features to consider

All work together with software or hardware that can convert text to speech

Some have mechanical-sounding speech, while others have high-quality, human-sounding speech

Some are software-based and need only a sound card or the sound hardware built into the computer plus speakers or headphones

Some plug into a slot inside the computer

Some connect to an external port on the computer

Most have adjustable volume

Most are equipped with an external jack for speakers or headphones

Some include settings for pitch or speaking voices (for example, male or female)

Some can define special pronunciation rules and add words to the synthesizer's dictionary

 Cost

Range: $0 (sound card bundled with computer)–1,200

Common: $125–750

242

___

Computer
Resources
for People
with
Disabilities

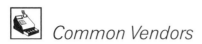 *Common Vendors*

Access Solutions

Artic Technologies

AT&T

Compusult Limited

Elan

GW Micro

IBM Corporation

Microsoft Corporation

Personal Data Systems, Inc.

Pulse Data

RC Systems

ScanSoft

 Additional information

To read text characters, speech synthesizers use special memory chips or software in which are stored thousands of rules the synthesizer uses to translate written text into speech. The translated text is known as *synthesized speech* (as opposed to *digitized speech*, which is recorded sound). A synthesizer can be either an external device that plugs into the computer (an external synthesizer) or a card that is put into a slot in the computer (an internal synthesizer). Many speech synthesizers are now software-based, generating speech sounds that go directly to a sound card or sound chip in the computer.

Macintosh: In Macintosh computer systems, speech synthesis is built in. Screen reading software for the blind or talking word processors for people with learning disabilities can take advantage of this built-in speech capability.

PCs: In computers running the various Windows operating systems, a separate software-based or hardware-based speech synthesizer is required for text-to-speech capability. Before purchasing a speech synthesizer for use with screen reading software for the blind or other talking programs, be sure that the synthesizer is compatible with the software to be used. It is also important that a sound card or sound chip in a computer can handle multiple streams of audio at the same time; for example, speech from the synthesizer while an MP3 file is playing. Be sure to consult with the vendor and computer salesperson to make sure your requirements are met. This is one area where it is recommended that you consult with a specialist in screen reading technology, a local group for the visually impaired, or an experienced user of this technology for help with purchase decisions.

 Related products

Note takers

Optical character recognition software and scanners

PDAs

Reading machines

Screen readers

Talking and large-print word processors

Screen Readers

A screen reader is a software program that works in conjunction with the computer's sound-processing hardware to provide verbalization of everything on the screen or output to a refreshable Braille display, including control buttons, menus, text, and punctuation.

 Use this tool to...

Provide access to print materials and manuals after they have been scanned into a computer

Provide auditory prompts and/or refreshable Braille-display output for access to menus and commands

Provide confirmation of keystrokes without looking at the screen

Make a computer accessible to someone with limited or no vision

 Potential users...

Need auditory feedback and/or refreshable Braille-display output to read text on the screen

Understand how to handle equipment but need print materials and manuals to be read aloud or displayed in refreshable Braille

Need auditory feedback and/or refreshable Braille-display output to navigate the screen and select commands

244

Computer
Resources
for People
with
Disabilities

 Features to consider

All can read units of text, such as characters, words, lines, and paragraphs

Some read selected portions of the screen either automatically or through commands from the keyboard

Some control the rate, pitch, and volume of speech output

Some use an external keypad or a touch tablet instead of or in addition to the regular keyboard to control screen reading functions, but most do not

Some employ artificial intelligence to make decisions about what the user wants spoken

All screen reader versions are compatible only with certain operating systems

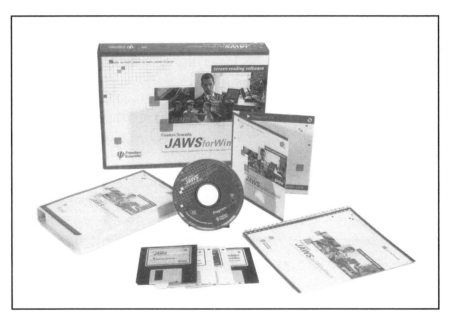

A screen reader reads printed material for people who have visual impairments. (Photo courtesy of FreedomScientific.com)

 Cost

Range: $300–1,200   Common: $595–1,200

Common vendors

American Printing House for the Blind, Inc.

Beyond Sight, Inc.

Dolphin Computer Access Limited

Freedom Scientific, Inc.

GW Micro

PulseData/HumanWare, Inc.

Reading Technologies

 Additional information

Macintosh: A screen reader designed for the Macintosh can use the built-in speech hardware to access Macintosh applications. It does not require an additional speech synthesizer.

PCs: Speech synthesizers are available in internal and external versions. Internal versions require a suitable expansion slot to be available in the computer; external versions require a free serial or parallel port compatible with the synthesizer. Check for compatibility of screen readers and speech synthesizers or cards when using MS-DOS or Windows operating systems. Some new programs create synthesized speech by using the sound card bundled with the computer when purchased (i.e., Sound Blaster or compatible).

 Related products

Optical character recognition and scanners

Reading machines

Speech synthesizers

Talking and large-print word processors

Screen Magnification Software

Screen magnification software may enlarge all or portions of the screen and usually contains a range of viewing preferences that the user can set.

 Use this tool to...

Magnify and/or modify the text and graphics on the screen

246

Computer
Resources
for People
with
Disabilities

 Potential users...

Need large text

Need to track cursor location

 Features to consider

Most include variable magnification levels (2x to 16x or more); some can provide levels of magnification between 1x and 2x

Most have a cursor that tracks the area being magnified or jumps to pop-up windows

Some include "cursor locator" functions that provide animation to draw the user's eye to the cursor location

Some offer split-screen viewing of magnified and unmagnified windows to magnify by line, selected segments, horizontal or vertical screens, and other windowing options

Some have optional speech-output capabilities

Some have advanced color-modification capabilities (e.g., the ability to set all backgrounds and all text to a specific color combination)

 Cost

Range: $0–595 (This product may be built into or bundled with another product at no additional cost.)

Common: $395 without speech output; $595 with speech output

 Common vendors

Ai Squared

Apple Computer, Inc.

Artic Technologies

Dolphin Computer Access

Freedom Scientific, Inc.

Innovation Management Group

Microsoft Corporation

Optelec USA, Inc.

Additional information

Screen magnification programs work best with application programs that do not use a large portion of the screen at one time. Programs with graphic images that stretch from one side of the screen to the other (or from the top to the bottom), such as games, will not work well with screen magnifiers in full-screen mode or at high levels of magnification, because the "zoom" window leaves out too much of the image. Programs with graphics that rapidly jump to different parts of the screen (e.g., web pages with animation) will also be difficult to use with screen magnification software.

Screen magnification software runs at the same time as other software programs are used. In some instances, this may cause compatibility problems with the operating system and application programs. Check with the manufacturer about any known conflicts.

Macintosh: Zoom, a screen magnifying utility, is included in the Macintosh System Software. This is a part of Universal Access, which is included on every Macintosh System CD, and replaces the CloseView utility, which was included with Macintosh System 9 and earlier. Zoom may or may not have been preinstalled on a computer, depending on purchase source.

PCs: Magnifier, a basic screen magnification program, is included with Windows 98 and later operating systems. It may be activated by using the Accessibility Wizard or by selecting it from Programs➡Accessories➡Accessibility. It may be used for short-term magnification needs, such as when installing more advanced magnification software. Compatibility issues involve the type of monitor, the version of operating system, and the software programs to be used with the screen magnification software.

 Related products

CCTVs

Monitor additions

Speech synthesizers

Talking and large-print word processors

ALTERNATE OUTPUT

248

Computer
Resources
for People
with
Disabilities

Monitor Additions

A monitor addition, or add-on, is any device that enhances or alters the use of a standard computer monitor.

Screen magnifiers fit over the screen of a computer monitor and magnify the images that appear on the screen.

Antiglare filters are clear screens that fit over a computer monitor screen and reduce glare and improve contrast. They also reduce ultraviolet rays and other energy emissions.

Monitor mounts come in a variety of styles and degrees of flexibility and allow adjustment of the monitor position.

 Use this tool to...

Screen magnifiers

Magnify the images of graphics or text on the monitor

Antiglare filters

Reduce glare from overhead lights and large windows

Reduce screen flicker

Increase the contrast on the monitor

Provide relief for some types of eye fatigue

Monitor mounts

Modify the position of the monitor to increase visibility

Accommodate many users of different heights or those in a prone or other nonstandard position

Accommodate users with visual field restrictions by placing the monitor in the most easily seen position

 Potential users...

Need low-level magnification to see the screen

Have sensitivity to bright light or work in areas of glare

Need increased clarity that can be created by reducing glare and/or increasing contrast

Need a monitor mount to position the screen closer or in a better viewing position

Need a monitor mount to operate the computer from a nonstandard position

 Features to consider

Screen magnifiers

Some are made to reduce distortion caused by magnification

Some include an antiglare polarizing filter and/or mounting hood to reduce room reflections and soften the light from the screen

Antiglare filters

Some include protection to reduce ELF and VLF electromagnetic energy

Some block damaging UVA and UVB rays to protect eyes from burning

Monitor mounts

All have a specific weight capacity

Some can move 360 degrees, tilt, or swivel

Some can be part of a table or can clamp to a table, be bolted down, or be attached to a wall or ceiling

 Cost

Screen magnifiers

Range: $160–250   Common: $200

Antiglare filters

Range: $10–200   Common: $50

Monitor mounts

Range: $50–800   Common: $50

 Common vendors

Screen magnifiers

Carolyn's Products for Enhanced Living

Florida New Concepts Marketing, Inc.

Grant Enterprises On Line/Safco-ErgoComfort Computer Accessories

250

Computer
Resources
for People
with
Disabilities

Antiglare filters

3M

DuPont Displays

Kensington Microware, Ltd.

Monitor mounts

Cables to Go

Esselte

Focused Technology

 Additional information

The products must fit the specific monitor being used.

 Related products

Screen magnification software

Augmentative and Alternative Communication Products (AAC)

An individual may choose to use electronic devices to augment or replace her or his voice. How people choose to communicate is an important and personal decision that involves both access issues and individual preference. Some preliminary information is provided here to introduce you to this field. We recommend that readers who are interested in assistive communication products bring together a team to carefully explore the range of products and their uses.

Computer-based systems: Computer-based communication devices use specific software integrated into a standard computer. Some software allows the display on the computer screen to change in response to the communicator's input. Computer-based systems are useful for communication as well as for typical computer applications, such as word processing, telecommunications, and limited environmental control. Depending on the individual's needs, additional hardware is usually required, such as an alternate keyboard, an alternate mouse, an electronic pointing device, or a single switch. This type of communication system can be installed on a desktop or a laptop computer, depending on how the system is designed.

Stand-alone or dedicated communication devices: Typically, stand-alone devices are portable and use digitized and/or synthesized speech. They are specifically designed for communicating and, because of their portability, are usually designed to be durable. Digitized communication devices use prerecorded speech for their messages. Synthesized communication devices use text translated into electronic speech. The messages on a system that uses synthesized speech can be picture based, word based, or text-to-speech based. Both digitized and synthesized systems are usually programmable and come in a wide variety of sizes and shapes, and with a wide variety of means of access. A small but growing number of these devices have the capacity to use both digitized and synthesized speech. As is the case with computer-based communication systems, some individuals, in order to meet their specific needs, may require additional hardware to operate a dedicated communication device. Such hardware may include a single switch, a joystick, a mouse, or an electronic pointing device. Many dedicated communication systems

252

Computer
Resources
for People
with
Disabilities

that offer digitized speech capabilities also include built-in infrared environ-mental controls for TVs, VCRs, and home automation devices. In addition, some systems that have digitized speech capabilities can also serve as an alternate keyboard or mouse on a computer. This feature can be used with infrared cordless access or through hard wiring to the computer. Some dedicated devices have a dynamic screen; others have a static screen.

 Use this tool to...

Communicate using specific software loaded on a commercially available desktop or laptop computer

Communicate using specific software loaded on a specially designed laptop computer

Communicate using a small, portable, dedicated communication device

Communicate using a small, portable device that can also be mounted, as needed, to wheelchairs

Communicate messages using short, digitized words, phrases, and sentences

Represent symbols, pictures, and objects with prerecorded messages

Change the content of messages on a dynamic basis

Create unique messages through picture, symbol, word, or text-based input

Create speech that may be specific to an individual's age, gender, and language

Clarify a message when the user's verbal communication is unintelligible

Present long messages, reports, and stories

Act as an alternate keyboard to a computer, as well as a communication system

 Potential users...

Require a method of communicating other than speech

Require support to communicate verbally

Benefit from using symbols, pictures, words, and/or text when communicating

Have speech patterns that are unintelligible

Features to consider

Some dedicated communication devices can be connected to a computer and used to replace the mouse and keyboard by functioning as a computer input device

Some devices are dedicated solely to communication

Some systems have vocabulary that is easily customized by the user or caregiver

Some devices use software with language-based symbol systems to create communication layouts

Some systems can be accessed through a variety of input devices, including touch screens, switches, alternate keyboards, mice, and alternative pointing devices

Some even have the capacity to provide input using Morse code

Many systems offer scanning options, including rate changes, pattern changes, and auditory scanning feedback

Many systems offer display options including color, black-and-white, and backlit screens

Some screens are very difficult to see outdoors in daylight (especially true with dynamic screens)

Many units vary in the quality of speech, depending on the type of synthesizer used

Some systems support both digitized speech and synthesized speech

Some systems can integrate a variety of functions into one unit, such as operating environmental controls, aids for daily living, and computer programs

Some systems can plug into a printer directly; a few have built-in printers

Some systems have a larger capacity for the size of messages that can be stored

Many systems are portable, but they vary in weight and size

Some vocabulary systems have the ability to store banks of phrases or messages for easy retrieval

Some systems use a language-based organization that uses symbols, pictures, words, and text-to-speech

254

Computer
Resources
for People
with
Disabilities

Some systems can be set to scan only spaces that contain messages, thereby speeding communication for a person scanning with single or double switches

Some devices provide auditory prompts, which make the system easier to use for a person with limited vision

Some systems can be set so that pressing blank spaces or unprogrammed keys will not provide any feedback or interrupt a sequence

 Cost

Computer-based systems

    Range: $300–25,000   Common: $3,000

Stand-alone or dedicated communication devices

    Range: $45–10,000   Common: $2,000–5,000

 Common vendors

AbleNet, Inc.

Adaptivation, Inc.

Applied Human Factors, Inc.

Assistive Technology, Inc.

Attainment Company, Inc.

Consultants for Communication Technology

Crestwood Company

Don Johnston, Inc.

DynaVox Systems (formerly Sentient Systems)

Enabling Devices and Toys for Special Children

Enkidu Research, Inc.

Franklin Electronic Publishers, Inc.

GEWA

The Great Talking Box Company

Gus Communications

Inclusive TLC, Inc.

LC Technologies

Luminaud, Inc.

Mayer-Johnson Company

Prentke Romich Company

Saltillo Corporation

TASH International, Inc.

Words+, Inc.

Zygo Industries, Inc.

 Additional information

When a consumer chooses a communication device, he or she is making a very important personal decision. During the selection process, it is very important to have a strong team in place that includes the individual, the family, educators, and specialists. Devices vary in the training required and the level of independent cognitive skills needed. A trial period with several devices may help eliminate costly mistakes.

Valuable sources of information about communication devices include:

United States Society for Augmentative and Alternative Communication (USSAAC)

Website: www.ussaac.org

International Society for Augmentative and Alternative Communication (ISAAC)

Website: www.isaac-online.org

AAC Institute

Website: www.aacinstitute.org

 Related products

Alternate keyboards

Electronic pointing devices

Electronic aids to daily living

Speech synthesizers

Switches and switch software

Touch screens

256

Computer
Resources
for People
with
Disabilities

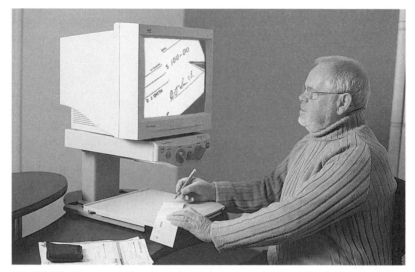

A CCTV video magnifier can enlarge a variety of materials, including maps and other print resources. (Photo courtesy of Pulse Data HumanWare, Inc.)

Closed-Circuit Televisions

Closed-circuit televisions (CCTVs) use a special television camera to magnify a printed page or another object that can be placed under the camera. The enlarged image is displayed on a monitor or television screen.

 Use this tool to...

Read print materials with the aid of magnification

Use magnification to assist with writing notes, letters, and other handwritten documents and with completing forms

Read information or see detail on objects

View text or objects at a distance

 Potential users...

Require large text

Benefit from greater contrast

Benefit from white text on a black background

Benefit from being able to select their own text and background color combinations

Benefit from seeing enlarged color detail in documents, such as maps, diagrams, and pictures

Benefit from an enlarged view of an object either nearby or at a distance

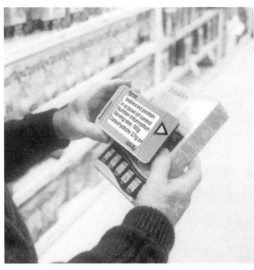

PocketViewer enlarges print 7 times on a small video screen and is ideal for reading menus in a restaurant, the TV Guide at home, the program in a concert hall, or the ingredients on a food box. (Photo courtesy of Pulse Data HumanWare, Inc.)

 Features to consider

All provide magnification of print materials

Most magnify in adjustable increments

Most are capable of reverse polarity, that is, displaying either a white image on a black background or a black image on a white background

Many have black-and-white screens

Some have color screens with selectable colors or full-color options

Some are handheld and portable

Some may be worn on the head or viewed with a screen mounted on glasses

Some can magnify objects or text at a distance, such as writing on a blackboard

Some can show an image on a computer screen and on the CCTV screen at the same time

258

Computer
Resources
for People
with
Disabilities

Some magnify output from a computer, calculator, chalkboard, white board, or even a microscope

 Cost

Range: $695–3,400   Common: $2,400

 Common vendors

Clarity

Enhanced Vision, Inc.

Optelec (Tieman) U.S.A., Inc.

OVAC Visual Systems

Pulse Data International, Ltd.

Sighted Electronics, Inc.

Telesensory

VideoEye! Corporation

Vision Technology, Inc

 Additional information

Text can be magnified up to 60 times on some units. The user normally moves, or "tracks," the item to be read under a fixed camera. With some portable units, a handheld camera is moved across the printed page. Many units automatically focus. Some units allow for objects to be viewed at a distance as well as up close.

 Related products

Monitor additions

Screen magnification software

Electronic Aids to Daily Living

An electronic aid to daily living (EADL) is used to control, from a remote location, electric appliances, telephones, and other items that typically plug into a wall outlet. Many such devices are also capable of emulating existing remote-control devices. EADLs were formerly called *environmental-control units.*

Use this tool to...

Turn on a computer system independently

Operate lamps, fans, stereos, intercoms, window blinds, and other household devices

Emulate handheld remote-control devices for televisions, entertainment systems, VCRs, CD-ROM players, etc.

Activate an emergency call button wired to a remote location in the building

Lock and unlock doors

Adjust a hospital bed independently

Activate a security system

 Potential users...

Need an alternative way to operate common devices and appliances

May use augmentative and alternative communication (AAC) systems

 Features to consider

Many control appliances plugged into an outlet

Some can control telephones

Some can control televisions, VCRs, stereo systems, and other devices with infrared remote control

Many may be activated by a single switch, using visual or auditory scanning, by voice recognition, by computer interface, or by timers

Some are dedicated, stand-alone devices; others are computer based

To control the various devices, most use either ultrasound, infrared, AC wiring built into the home, or radio frequency

Many have the option to control a single device, several devices, or a great many devices

Some AAC devices include EADL functions

 Cost

Range: $50–7,500 (with AAC devices)

Common: basic functions $300; advanced functions $4,500

260

Computer
Resources
for People
with
Disabilities

 Common vendors

AbleNet, Inc.

Applied Future Technologies, Inc.

Consultants for Communication Technology

Dynavox Systems

GenesisOne Technologies Incorporated

GEWA

Gus Communications

InterAct Plus

Madentec, Ltd.

Med Labs Inc.

Prentke Romich Company

Quartet Technology, Inc.

TASH International, Inc.

Enabling Devices and Toys for Special Children

Words+, Inc.

X-10 (USA), Inc.

Zygo Industries, Inc.

 Additional information

Some EADLs can be purchased as a software package to be used on a personal computer; others are stand-alone devices. EADL software is available for both Macintosh and PCs, but requires additional hardware interfaces. To use these devices with a single switch, you need an additional interface.

 Related products

Interface devices

Switches and switch software

Voice recognition systems

Note Takers

Two types of note takers are frequently used as assistive technology. The first type, which is generally marketed as a mainstream product, is a lightweight device with a built-in word processor and possibly other applications. It permits text to be entered, stored, and transferred to a printer (via infrared) or computer (via cable). It can serve as a useful alternative to handwriting for individuals with physical or learning disabilities. Realizing this, manufacturers are starting to add standard or optional assistive features, such as key-repeat rate adjustment and word prediction.

The other type of note taker is specifically designed for people who are blind. These are portable units that employ either a Braille keyboard or a standard keyboard to allow the user to enter information. Text is stored in files that can be read and edited using the built-in speech synthesizer or Braille display. Files may be sent to a printer or Braille embosser, or transferred to a computer. Increasingly, these types of note takers also include additional applications, such as calendars, Internet browsers, address books, and other utilities.

 Use this tool to...

Take notes in class, meetings, or conferences

Access the Internet by connecting to a phone line or Ethernet connection

Send and receive e-mail by connecting to a phone line or Ethernet connection

Instruct in writing and reading Braille

 Potential users...

Users with handwriting difficulties

Prefer or have an easier time typing notes, rather than writing them by hand

Need a more portable, more accessible, or more economical alternative to a laptop computer

People who are blind

Read and write in Braille

Need a way to take notes and be able to transfer them to a computer

Need an electronic method for keeping track of appointments, contact information, etc.

262

Computer
Resources
for People
with
Disabilities

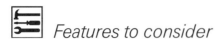 *Features to consider*

Most have text-editing capability

Most can read/write to Microsoft Word files

Some permit additional applications to be added

Most include a calculator, calendar, or other utilities

Some can connect to the Internet

Some can send and receive e-mail

Most can print using conventional printers

For users with handwriting difficulties

Most include some access utilities for users with physical disabilities

Some permit the addition of word prediction or other utilities for users with learning disabilities

For people who are blind

Some allow information to be entered in Braille

Most can be purchased with either a standard or Braille keyboard

Most have built-in speech synthesizers

Most can accommodate headphones to permit private listening

Most can turn auditory feedback on or off

Some include an appointment book, which can sound a tone to remind the user of scheduled appointments

Most can print using Braille embossers

Some have refreshable Braille displays

Some can produce eight-dot Braille

Some can also function as a cell phone

 Cost

Users with handwriting difficulties

Range: $200–$700   Common: $200

People who are blind

Range: $1,000–7,000   Common: $3,500

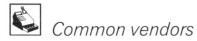 *Common vendors*

Users with handwriting difficulties

AlphaSmart, Inc.

Branium Technologies, Inc.

People who are blind

AlphaSmart, Inc.

American Printing House for the Blind, Inc.

Freedom Scientific, Inc.

PulseData/HumanWare, Inc.

 Additional Information

Generally, note takers are limited in functionality when compared to a laptop or desktop computer because of their processor design and limited memory and storage capacity. However, they do have the advantage of long battery life and portability.

 Related products

Screen readers

Speech synthesizers

Reading machines

Braille embossers and translators

Refreshable Braille displays

PDAs

Reading Machines

A reading machine transforms printed material into an electronic data format that is read aloud by a speech synthesizer. It consists of three forms of technology: a scanner to convert a print document into electronic format, an optical character recognition (OCR) program to convert the document into computer text, and text-to-speech (TTS) technology to read the text aloud using speech synthesis. Reading machines may be stand-alone systems, like a desktop unit or something as small as a writing pen, or may be a computer

264

Computer
Resources
for People
with
Disabilities

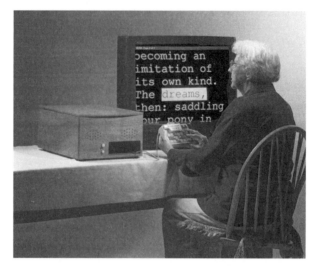

*With VERA, a reading machine, any printed material
can be converted to an electronic format, allowing
you to read books, magazines, and even junk mail.
(Photo courtesy of FreedomScientific.com)*

modified by the addition of a scanner, OCR software, and screen reading software.

 ## Use this tool to...

Read books, mail, business documents, and faxed information

Improve reading comprehension by listening to materials being read as they are displayed on the computer screen

Read isolated words that are difficult to decipher

Avoid eyestrain when reading lengthy materials

 ## Potential users...

Have vision impairments, including low vision or total blindness

Have learning disabilities affecting their ability to read

Need print materials read aloud

 ## Features to consider

All have speech output

All use a scanner

Some have a document feeder for the scanner

Some are handheld

Some provide synonyms or definitions for scanned words

Most automatically determine page orientation

Most recognize many typeface styles

Most can handle multicolumn pages

Most recognize a variety of print qualities

Some are compact for greater portability

Some are specially designed to more easily accommodate books

Some support Braille or large-print output

Some read faxed documents

Some control scanning and reading functions with a computer keyboard, a separate keypad, or a joystick

Some show an actual view of the scanned document

Some offer options for highlighting by word, sentence, and paragraph

 Cost

To upgrade an existing computer

Range: $250–2,000

Common: $750–1,500

Stand-alone machines

Range: $300–3,500

Common: $3,000

 Common vendors

BAUM Retec AG

Freedom Scientific, Inc

JBliss Imaging Systems

Kurzweil Educational Systems

Premier Assistive Technology

Pulse Data/Humanware, Inc.

Robotron Group

266

Computer
Resources
for People
with
Disabilities

Schamex Research

Telesensory, Inc.

Wizcom

Xerox Imaging Systems, Inc.

 Additional information

Macintosh: Although there are no reading-system software packages for Macintosh computers that are specifically designed for people who are blind, there are several OCR systems that can be used with a scanner and a screen reader to give people with visual disabilities access to printed material using a Macintosh computer.

PCs: A reading machine is a unique combination of several access products. If you are modifying a standard computer so it can also be used as a reading machine, you will need to be certain that all the hardware and software components are compatible. Read the software package carefully for compatibility information about the scanner and speech synthesizer required, as well as the computer system requirements, such as amount of memory needed.

 Related products

Note takers

Optical character recognition and scanners

Screen readers

Speech synthesizers

Wireless Products (Cell Phones, Pagers, GPS)

Wireless devices, such as cell phones, pagers, and GPS receivers, are used by people all over the world to help them communicate and travel more easily and safely. Thanks to improved accessibility, people with disabilities can now enjoy the benefits of these products.

A cell phone, or cellular phone, is a portable telephone that uses radio transmissions to communicate either with users of the public telephone network or with other cell phone users. The coverage area of a cell phone network is divided into small segments, or cells, containing a radio transmitter and receiver. As a user moves through the coverage area, the cell phone's signal is automatically routed to the cell with the best reception. There are numerous cell phone networks around the world, and a cell phone's specifications must match the networks on which it is intended to operate. Cell phones come in many different styles and sizes, and their features range from simple telephone functions to the capabilities found in a PDA (personal digital assistant).

A pager is a small telecommunication device that is designed to alert the user with either a beep or a vibration that a phone call needs to be returned or a message requires attention. Simple one-way pagers are receive-only devices that display a telephone number and numeric codes that correspond to specific messages for the user. These pagers can be as small as a wristwatch and are typically carried in a shirt pocket or clipped to a belt. More sophisticated one-way pagers can display short text messages. Two-way pagers are also available that can both transmit and receive messages and simple graphics. They are typically about the size of a pocket calculator and have a small keyboard and display screen large enough to accommodate several lines of text.

The GPS (global positioning system) consists of 24 satellites positioned in orbit around the earth so that four satellites are always above the horizon. A GPS receiver on the ground that is able to receive radio signals from three of the satellites can, under optimum conditions, pinpoint the user's location to within 15 feet. Reception of the fourth satellite can also give altitude data. Military GPS receivers are capable of even greater accuracy. A GPS receiver can display location information either as latitude and longitude or as a position on a map, depending on the sophistication of the receiver. GPS receivers are used by outdoor enthusiasts while pursuing cross-country activities and in automobile navigation systems that can guide the driver to a particular location and provide turn-by-turn directions and an estimated time of arrival. GPS navigation systems for the blind have been developed that provide orientation information while the user is walking, riding in an automobile, or on public transportation.

 Use these tools to...

Cell phones

> Make and receive phone calls when away from a regular phone

> Send and receive text messages

> Send and receive multimedia messages

> Send and receive pictures

> Keep track of daily schedules

> Store address-book information

> Play games

> Browse the Internet

268

Computer
Resources
for People
with
Disabilities

Pagers

Be alerted that a phone call needs to be returned

Be alerted to a message that requires attention

Answer a message from another pager or from a computer

Initiate a message to another pager or to a computer

GPS

Determine your location while walking

Determine your location while riding in an automobile or on public transportation

Plan a route to a location

Be guided to a location

Retrace the route back to your starting point

Find points of interest in your vicinity

Learn the distance to a location

 Potential users...

Cell phones

Are often away from a regular phone

Use a cell phone to replace a regular phone

Use the PDA functions included in full-featured cell phones

Find it difficult to locate or use a pay phone

Pagers

Need to stay in touch but do not have a phone available at all times

Need to send and receive text messages

Need to communicate but cannot use a cell phone effectively because of a hearing disability

GPS

Need to know their location while participating in cross-country activities

Need location information and driving directions while traveling

Are blind people who enjoy walking independently in unfamiliar areas

Are blind people who want to know their location while riding in an automobile or on public transportation

Are blind people who want to help with driving directions while traveling with others

 Features to consider

Cell phones

All make and receive phone calls wirelessly

Many have selectable ring tones

Some can use Short Message Service, a type of text-based communication

Some can send and receive Multimedia Messaging Service, which allows sharing of documents, sound recordings, or movie clips

Some can surf the Web

Some include games

Some offer PDA features, such as an appointment calendar, an address book, and note taking

Some have speech output when access software is loaded

Some have both speech output and a Braille display

Pagers

All can receive a page alert signal

Many can alert the user with either a beep or vibration

All can display the phone number of a call that needs to be returned

Most can display codes for preprogrammed messages

Some can display full text messages

Some can both send and receive messages

Some can send the user messages that were missed while the pager was off or out of range

Some can perform additional services, such as sending faxes, TTY chatting, surfing the Web, getting stock quotes, and organizing daily tasks

Some can speak the information on the display

GPS

All can give the user information about geographic location

Some display location information in latitude and longitude

270

Computer
Resources
for People
with
Disabilities

Most can pinpoint the user's location on a map

Some GPS receivers are stand-alone units

Some GPS receivers connect to PDAs that run map software

Some GPS receivers are integrated with PDAs to provide speech and/or Braille output to help a person who is blind with orientation and navigation

 Cost

Cell phones

Range: $0 (with service plan)–450

Common: $100

Pagers

Range: $0 (with service plan)–300

Common: $55

GPS

Range: $100–1,600

Common: $250 (commercial market); $1,000 (assistive-technology market)

 Common vendors

Cell phones

AT&T

Cellular One

Cingular

Nextel

Speech and Braille Unlimited

Sprint

SunCom

Tek-Talk

T-Mobile

Verizon

Pagers

CPR Technology

DeafNation

Motorola

Research in Motion

Wynd Communications Corporation

YoMax Communications

GPS

Freedom Scientific, Inc.

Garmin International, Inc.

Pulse Data/Humanware, Inc.

Thales Navigation

VisuAide

 Additional information

Cell phones are available from a wide variety of sources, including service providers. When purchased through service providers with an appropriate service plan, they are often free after rebate; in some cases the buyer even comes out ahead. While shopping around for the best deal, however, it must be kept in mind that the phone is only as good as the coverage in the area of intended operation.

In the past, blind people were unable to use the advanced features of cell phones because of the lack of any type of useful feedback. However, it is now possible to access these features on some models of cell phones because of software developed by Code Factory in Spain and Brand & Gröber Communications GbR in Germany. The phones supported thus far are running the Symbian operating system, but other operating systems will be supported in the future. In addition to these cell phones being made accessible through the creation of special software, there is also an accessible cell phone with speech and Braille output that includes many of the functions of a PDA.

Access to cell phones by people who use hearing aids has been very limited due to incompatibility issues between cell phones and hearing aids. New requirements established by the Federal Communications Commission require cell phone manufacturers to address the needs of people with hearing impairments in the near future. Be sure to inquire about compatibility with hearing aids before purchasing a cell phone.

272

Computer
Resources
for People
with
Disabilities

Like cell phones, pagers are often free with a service plan or after a rebate. How well a pager will work in a particular coverage area must be considered at the time of purchase. A potential user must also consider whether a simple one-way pager or a full-featured, two-way pager with all the bells and whistles is needed. Finally, if travel to other parts of the country is anticipated, the pager and service plan should be chosen accordingly.

Two-way text pagers have become popular for communication by deaf and hard-of-hearing people who are unable to use a cell phone effectively. In addition to text messaging, pagers can offer other features, such as sending faxes, TTY chat, web browsing, and personal organizational tools.

Individuals who are blind can benefit from pagers with speech output. One such pager speaks the phone number of the caller and the time of the call. The user can then hold the pager next to the mouthpiece of a touch-tone phone, press a button, and have the pager produce tones to dial the number.

GPS navigation can be done by using a stand-alone handheld receiver, adding a receiver and software to a PDA or using a system built into a vehicle. Stand-alone GPS receivers are impractical for people who are blind or visually impaired because of their small display size and lack of speech output. However, packages including a receiver and software are now available for PDAs with speech and Braille output, making it possible to use GPS for orientation and navigation. A dedicated GPS navigation system also exists that consists of a standard PDA that runs specially written speech output and mapping software combined with a GPS receiver.

 Related products

Braille displays

Note takers

PDAs

Screen readers

PDAs

A PDA (personal digital assistant) is a small handheld computer that has calendar, address book, and note-taking functions. Sophisticated PDAs can include Web-browsing, e-mail, and office applications. Data can be input either via a small keyboard or with a stylus and touch-sensitive pad or screen. PDAs run on proprietary operating systems or on other common operating systems, such as Windows CE.

Use this tool to...

Keep track of your daily schedule

Store addresses and phone numbers

Take notes

Browse the Web

Send and receive e-mail

Perform office tasks using abbreviated versions of business application software

Augment or replace the voice when communicating

 Potential users...

Need the functions provided by a PDA, but do not need the full functionality of a laptop computer

Need a longer battery life and better portability than that provided by a laptop computer

Need a combination PDA and augmentative/alternative communication device

Need a dedicated augmentative/alternative communication device that can be funded through Medicare and is small, lightweight, and portable

 Features to consider

Some have a small keyboard for input

Some have a touch-sensitive screen or pad for input with a stylus

All have a calendar, an address book, and note-taking functions

Some have e-mail functions

Some have Web-browsing functions

Some have a media player

Some can connect to computers or other PDAs either via a cable or with infrared or Bluetooth

Some can connect to cell phones

Some have ports for modem, Ethernet, and memory cards

Some can run abbreviated versions of office applications

274

Computer
Resources
for People
with
Disabilities

Some can act only as a dedicated augmentative/alternative communication device

Some can act as both an augmentative/alternative communication device and a PDA

Some are voice activated and offer speech output

 Cost

Range: $250–6,000   Common: $2,700

 Common vendors

Enkidu Research

Freedom Scientific, Inc.

Hewlett-Packard

Independent Living Aids, Inc.

LS & S

MaxiAids

Parrot

Pulse Data/HumanWare, Inc.

Saltillo Corporation

 Additional information

PDAs that are generally available on the commercial market cannot be used effectively by people with disabilities that prevent them from using a small keyboard or stylus for input or a small screen for output. In the assistive-technology market, many adaptive PDAs have been developed, ranging from small, pocket-sized organizers that record notes, appointment schedules, and address book information in a person's own voice to sophisticated devices that have speech and Braille output and offer many of the functions of a laptop or desktop computer. Many PDAs can connect to computers or other PDAs, either via a cable or wirelessly, and can communicate with the rest of the world with either a built-in modem or cellular phone connection. Cell phones that include PDA functions are available on the commercial market and can now be made accessible through the addition of speech-output software. The addition of augmentative/alternative communication software and other modifications can enable a PDA to augment or replace a person's voice.

Related products

Augmentative and alternative communication products

Braille displays

Note takers

Screen readers

Speech synthesizers

Wireless products

TTYs and TTY Modems

A teletypewriter (TTY), or telecommunication device for the deaf (TDD), is a device with a keyboard that sends and receives typed messages over a telephone line. If a person lacks access to a TTY but has access to a computer, online relay services are available that will place a TTY call for that individual. The website www.sprintrelayonline.com will connect the computer user with a relay operator.

A TTY modem is a Weitbrecht/Baudot–compatible modem for a personal computer. Standard modems use ASCII code to communicate over phone lines; TTY modems use Baudot code at a fixed baud rate of 45. A standard modem generally cannot communicate with a TTY, although some TTYs allow the user to select either Baudot or ASCII code at up to 300 baud. A compatible voice modem with digital signal processing (v.253 compatible) will communicate with a TTY with the appropriate software.

Some internal modems are voice compatible and can be used with SoftTTY or myTTY software to perform Baudot communication. These modems are standard in Macs with G3 processors.

 Use this tool to...

Call other TTY users

Call a relay system that will read your TTY message to the standard phone user whom you would like to call

Connect with TTY automated services, such as a bank

 Potential users...

Cannot talk and/or hear and require text in order to communicate by telephone

276

Computer
Resources
for People
with
Disabilities

Want to communicate with another person who uses a TTY for telephone communication

 Features to consider

A TTY may be portable, desktop, or personal-computer based

All TTYs have a display that shows the message as it is entered or received

Some TTYs include built-in printers

Some TTYs offer various options for the display, such as color, text size, and direction of scrolling

Some TTYs are compatible with Braille devices

Some TTYs have a large visual display for individuals with vision issues

Some TTYs offer speed dialing

Some TTYs have a built-in ring flasher

Some TTYs feature voice carryover, which allows one party to speak directly to the other while the return messages are typed and appear on the screen

Some TTYs and TTY modems allow storage of conversations for later review

Some TTYs and TTY modems can answer automatically with programmable messages and can record incoming messages

Some TTY modems can automatically adjust to receive from either a TTY or another computer

All TTY modems require telecommunication software

 Cost

TTYs

> Range: $200–900
>
> Common: $400

TTY modems

> Range: $150–400
>
> Common: $200

TTY software

> Range: $80–300
>
> Common: $90

Common Vendors

TTYs

> Ameriphone, Inc.
>
> AT&T Accessible Communication Products
>
> DeafWorks
>
> HARC Mercantile, Ltd.
>
> Harris Communications, Inc.
>
> Hear More, Inc.
>
> HITEC Group International
>
> LS&S, LLC
>
> Phone TTY, Inc.
>
> Potomac Technology
>
> SSK Technology, Inc.
>
> Telesensory
>
> Ultratec
>
> WCI Technology

TTY modems and software

> AT&T Wireless Services Messaging Division
>
> Harris Communications, Inc.
>
> Institute for Disabilities Research and Training, Inc.
>
> Intelligent Products
>
> Microflip, Inc.
>
> NXI Communicators
>
> Phone-TTY, Inc.
>
> Wynd Communications

 Additional information

Wireless communications: Cellular and cordless phones can connect to some portable TTYs. Some pagers can send and receive TTY messages and e-mails and send faxes; some feature the capability to support live TTY chats. Some pagers can send a text-to-speech message and send a text message to any

278

Computer
Resources
for People
with
Disabilities

one-way alphanumeric pager. Some text pagers can send text-to-speech messages to any telephone in the form of a computerized voice.

Voice carryover: A person with a hearing loss who has a good speaking voice can use a voice-carryover phone to communicate with another party. The individual would use his or her own voice to speak to the other party, while a relay operator would key in the party's response for the person with hearing loss to read on their LCD screen.

Hearing carryover: A person with an inability to speak but with the ability to hear can use a TTY to type his or her responses for a relay operator to read to a second party. The second party can then speak at a normal rate directly to the first party. This enables the person with the speech disability to directly hear the voice of the person he or she is communicating with.

 Related products

Assistive listening devices

Assistive technology for the deaf and hard of hearing

PDAs

Wireless products

Assistive Listening Devices

A person with a hearing loss may encounter frustrations while talking to people one-on-one and in groups. It is also difficult for people with hearing loss to participate in lectures, performances, classes, and church services. Assistive listening devices (ALDs) are used to amplify the speaker's voice to a level where the person with hearing loss can hear more clearly. The device generally involves a transmitter with a microphone for the speaker. It transmits an FM or an infrared signal to a receiver that the person with hearing loss accesses using headphones, ear buds, or a neck loop.

 Use this tool to...

Participate in numerous activities, such as:
classes
lectures
theater performances
movies
worship services
business meetings

small group discussions
one-on-one conversations
listening to television

 Potential users...

Need target sounds enhanced in order to participate in a group

Use hearing aids in conjunction with a neck loop

May not use hearing aids but may benefit from getting auditory feedback by using headphones or an ear bud

 Features to consider

Some ALDs have a microphone built into the receiver and are used for one-on-one and small group conversations

Some ALDs can be used with multiple receivers and one transmitter so that several people with hearing loss can participate in the same event

Some ALDs feature noise-canceling microphones to block out distracting noises

Some ALDs can be used with a conference microphone for meetings or group discussions

Some receivers include environmental microphones that can be used along with the microphone on the transmitter, enabling people to hear contributions from audience members

Some ALDs are wired into a large sound system, such as a movie theater or performance auditorium

Some ALDs use FM signal, and some use infrared signal

Some ALDs can be wired through a television to improve sound without disturbing other viewers

Some ALDs can be wired into cars, through bank-teller microphones, and into small rooms so that a hearing-aid wearer with a telecoil, or T-coil, has immediate access to sound amplification by flipping the T-switch on the back of their hearing aid

 Cost

Range: $25–915   Common: $500

SPECIALIZED PRODUCTS

280

Computer
Resources
for People
with
Disabilities

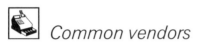 *Common vendors*

ALDs, Inc.

Direct Ear

Echo Tech

Harris Communications

Hear More

HiTech

LS&S, LLC

Mega Ear

Potomac Technology

Siemans

Turbo Ear

Williams Sound

 Additional information

Hearing aids equipped with a T-coil benefit from access to numerous technologies associated with ALDs. The access is far more direct and easy to use. If a person has T-coils in her hearing aids, she can use neck loops and silhouettes to hear TVs, stereos, telephones, answering machines, or infrared and FM systems. A T-coil is an accessory on a hearing aid that must be requested specifically by the consumer.

Assistive listening devices work well for people with certain kinds of hearing loss. They are not effective for everyone. A person with severe to profound hearing loss may benefit from an ALD. Depending on the type of hearing loss, some people with more moderate hearing loss can hear the amplification but do not gain clarity and thus choose not to use an ALD. Some can benefit from the device but dislike the limitation of only hearing the person wearing the microphone and not other people in the room.

 Related products

Assistive technology for the deaf and hard of hearing

TTYs and TTY modems

Although technically not an assistive-technology device, a Speech-to-Speech relay service certainly provides technology-related help to people with speech disabilities, taking advantage of existing telephone technology in a very valuable way.

Speech-to-Speech service provides human "revoicers" for people who have difficulty being understood on the telephone. It is the only way for many people to telephone others who are unaccustomed to their speech. The FCC requires all states to provide Speech-to-Speech services. If you have a speech disability, you can dial toll-free to reach a patient, trained operator who is familiar with many speech patterns and has acute hearing. The operator makes telephone calls for you and repeats your words exactly. Speech-to-Speech service is currently available 24 hours a day in all states.

Many Speech-to-Speech users have Parkinson's disease, cerebral palsy, multiple sclerosis, or muscular dystrophy. Other users include people who stutter, have ALS, or have had a laryngectomy. The service is also helpful for individuals who use a speech synthesizer. You can try the service, report problems, or get more information by calling (800) 854-7784 and asking for Dr. Bob Segalman (in the communication assistant's directory).

For a list of Speech-to-Speech access numbers in the United States, go to: www.stsnews.com/RelayNews/STSDialUpTelnumbers.html

You can also access STS by dialing 711 and asking for Speech-to-Speech.

Australia also provides Speech-to-Speech Relay (SSR). Contact: Bobbie Blackson at feedback@aceinfo.net.au.

Sweden has just extended its STS trial for one year. Contact: Birgit G. Lindh at birgit.g.lindh@telia.com. Tel. +0046-175-623-68.

Assistive Technology for the Deaf and Hard of Hearing

Assistive technology for deaf and hard-of-hearing people bridges the gap of communication. The various technologies currently available enhance communication across a range of environments, from phone use to classroom access. Below is a brief description of some of the available technologies.

282

———

Computer
Resources
for People
with
Disabilities

Alert systems

People with hearing loss may be unable to hear sounds, such as a ringing telephone, a doorbell, a smoke alarm, an alarm clock, or a baby crying. Alert systems work in conjunction with lights and tactile alerts to notify a person of such environmental noises. For example, if the doorbell were to ring, a light would flash. Or an alarm clock would trigger a bed shaker to awaken the user. Some alert systems feature several options built into one unit; other systems require items to be purchased separately to build the package. Some are hardwired and some are wireless. The systems can be used in schools, workplaces, and other public areas to flash a light for the signaling of bells or emergency alarms.

Telephone amplifiers

Amplifiers for people with hearing loss can be connected to an existing phone through an in-line amplifier or a slip-on device that covers the listening portion of the handset. Alternatively, some phones can be purchased with an amplifier already built in. Telephone amplifiers include a volume toggle to increase or decrease the amplification level. Some have the ability to change the tone to accommodate an individual's hearing-frequency loss.

Hearing aids

Hearing aids continue to improve as the technology develops. Although the price of hearing aids is high, newer aids offer many more benefits than mere amplification. Digital hearing aids filter the sound so its quality is improved based on the user's specific requirements. In addition, a T-coil can be added to most hearing aids. A T-coil is a very important tool; it provides access to many devices, some of which are described above. With a T-coil or T-switch, the individual can use a neck loop that can plug into any device with a standard jack, including listening devices, Walkmans, and some newer phones and answering machines. It also allows the user to talk on the phone without removing her or his hearing aid.

Text pagers

Text-to-text pagers have become popular for people with hearing loss. Some of the newer models work much like a portable TTY; they can not only send text to another pager, but can also send a text-to-speech message to a phone, creating a computer voice to speak the text. Currently, the companies Wyndtell, T Mobile, and AT&T are leading the market, although service is not available in all areas as of this publication.

Captioning

Closed captioning is defined as visible text for spoken audio. Closed captioning makes it possible for people who have difficulty hearing or understanding spoken words to read them on the television screen. It is a feature that is required by law to be built into any television made after 1988. A caption decoder can be used with a television that does not have built-in captioning. Most current television shows, movies, and live news broadcasts offer captioning. Some emergency broadcasts, however, may not have captioning. Captioning is used by people with hearing loss or deafness in their homes; it is also used in noisy environments, like restaurants, airports, or in other circumstances when sound is a barrier.

Real-time captioning is performed by a person with a transcription device. He or she transcribes the spoken dialog of meetings or lectures, projecting it either onto a laptop that sits directly in front of the person with hearing loss or onto a screen for the entire group to read.

Video conferencing/remote interpreting

Video conferencing is becoming more popular in the deaf community. With the use of a high-speed Internet connection and a Web cam, people can use sign language to communicate long distance. Because of a growing shortage of qualified sign-language interpreters, some agencies are moving toward this option for interpreter services. An interpreter can stay in one place and use cameras and audio input to interpret for a deaf person at a different location. This enables the interpreter to cover more assignments in one day. Video conferencing has also become useful for meetings and conferences as teleconferences have become more popular. The technology allows people from many different locations who use interpreters to attend the same meeting.

For people who have a high-speed Internet connection and a Web cam at home, video-relay services, such as those provided by AT&T and Sprint, are available to use instead of a TTY. This is very useful since sign language is often a more natural form of communication than written English.

Websites

www.relaycall.com/vrs

www.usavrs.com

www.sorensonvrs.com

Manufacturers

Ameriphone, Inc.

284

Computer
Resources
for People
with
Disabilities

Sonic Alert, Inc.

Silent Call Communications

Ultratec

Walker Equipment

Common vendors

Harris Communications

LS&S, LLC

Maxi Aids

Potomac Technologies

Part III

Helpful Resources and References

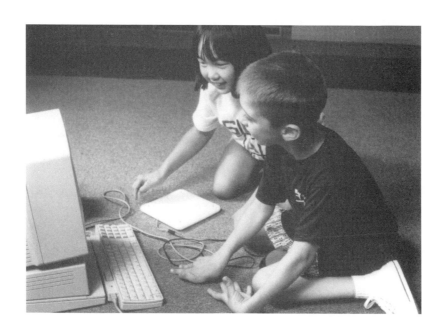

Contents

Part III contains lists of key references and resources to point you in appropriate directions for getting started on your search for assistive technology. In some cases the value of a given resource will be to lead you to other resources, especially if you are contacting sources via the Internet. By following up on some of the national references listed here, you should be able to identify resources and contacts in your own community, which, of course, is the main goal. The references and resources are organized into the following sections:

287

Alliance for
Technology
Access
Resource
Centers

Alliance for Technology Access Resource Centers

The Alliance for Technology Access is a growing network, with new members joining regularly. If you are interested in becoming a member of the ATA, please contact us for guidelines and an application, or visit our website.

The contact information for ATA members changes from time to time. For the most up-to-date information, visit our website or call our office.

Alliance for Technology Access (main office)

1304 Southpoint Blvd., Suite 240 (707) 778-3011
Petaluma CA 94954 (707) 778-3015, TTY
E-mail: ATAinfo@ATAccess.org (707) 765-2080, fax
Website: www.ATAccess.org

Resource Centers

Alabama

Technology Assistance for Special Consumers (T.A.S.C.)

PO Box 443, 915 Monroe St. (256) 532-5996
Huntsville AL 35804 (256) 532-2355, fax
E-mail: tasc@hiwaay.net
Website: http://tasc.ataccess.org

Arizona

Technology Access Center of Tucson, Inc. (TACT)

4710 East 29th St. (520) 745-5588, ext. 1265
Tucson AZ 85711 (520) 790-7637, fax
Mailing address: PO Box 13178
Tuscon AZ 85732
E-mail: tactaz@aol.com
Website: www.ed.arizona.edu/tact/index.htm

Arkansas

Technology Resource Center

c/o Arkansas Easter Seal Society (501) 227-3600
3920 Woodland Heights Rd. (501) 227-3601, fax
Little Rock AR 72212-2495
E-mail: atrce@aol.com
Website: www.iser.com/easterseal-AR.html

288

Computer
Resources
for People
with
Disabilities

California

Center for Accessible Technology (CforAT)
2547 8th St., 12-A
Berkeley CA 94710-2572
E-mail: info@cforat.org
Website: www.cforat.org

(510) 841-3224
(510) 841-5621, TTY
(510) 841-7956, fax

Computer Access Center
6234 West 87th St.
Los Angeles CA 90045
Mailing address: PO Box 5336
Santa Monica CA 90409-5336
E-mail: info@cac.org
Website: www.cac.org

(310) 338-1597
(310) 338-9318, fax

iTECH Center at Parents Helping Parents
3041 Olcott St.
Santa Clara CA 95054-3222
E-mail: iTech@php.com
Website: www.php.com

(408) 727-5775
(408) 727-0182, fax

Kern Assistive Technology Center
3101 N. Sillect Ave., Suite 101
Bakersfield CA 93308
E-mail: katc2003@sbcglobal.net

(661) 852-3399
(661) 852-3336, TTY
(661) 324-0463, fax

San Diego Assistive Technology Center
United Cerebral Palsy Association
6153 Fairmount Ave., Suite 150
San Diego CA 92120
E-mail: ucpsdatc@pacbell.net

(858) 278-5420
(619) 325-7135, fax

Team of Advocates for Special Kids (TASK)
100 W. Cerritos Ave.
Anaheim CA 92805-6546
E-mail: taskca@aol.com
Website: www.taskaca.org

(714) 533-8275
(714) 533-2533, fax

Florida

CITE, Lighthouse for the Visually Impaired
215 E. New Hampshire St.
Orlando FL 32804
E-mail: citeinfo@cite-fl.com
Website: www.centralfloridalighthouse.org

(407) 898-2483
(407) 895-5255, fax

Georgia

TechAble, Inc.
1114 Brett Dr., Suite 100
Conyers GA 30094
E-mail: techweb@techable.net
Website: www.techable.org

(770) 922-6768, voice, TTY
(770) 922-6769, fax

289

Alliance for
Technology
Access
Resource
Centers

Hawaii

Aloha Special Technology Access Center (ALOHA STAC)
710 Green St.
Honolulu HI 96813
E-mail: astachi@yahoo.com
Website: www.geocities.com/astachi

(808) 523-5547
(808) 536-3765, fax

Idaho

United Cerebral Palsy of Idaho, Inc. (UCP Idaho)
5420 West Franklin Rd., Suite A
Boise ID 83706
E-mail: info@ucpidaho.org
Website: www.ucpidaho.org

(888) 289-3259
(208) 377-8070
(208) 322-7133, fax

Illinois

Northern Illinois Center for Adaptive Technology (NICAT)
3615 Louisiana Rd.
Rockford IL 61108-6195
E-mail: davegrass@earthlink.net
Website: http://nicat.ataccess.org

(815) 229-2163
(815) 229-2135, fax

Indiana

Assistive Technology Training and Information Center (ATTIC)
A Resource Center for Independent Living
1721 Washington Ave.
Vincennes IN 47591
E-mail: inattic1@aol.com
Website: www.theattic.org

(800) 96-ATTIC (962-8842)
(812) 886-0575
(812) 886-1128, fax

Kansas

Technology Resource Solutions for People
1710 West Schilling Rd.
Salina KS 67401
E-mail: kreed@occk.com
Website: www.occk.com/trsp.htm

(800) 526-9731
(785) 827-9383
(785) 827-7051, TTY
(785) 823-2015, fax

290

Computer
Resources
for People
with
Disabilities

Kentucky

Bluegrass Technology Center (BTC)
961 Beasley St., Suite 103A
Lexington KY 40509
E-mail: office@bluegrass-tech.org
Website: www.bluegrass-tech.org

(859) 294-4343
(800) 209-7767, in state
(859) 294-0704, fax

EnTech: Enabling Technologies of Kentuckiana
Louisville Free Public Library
301 York St.
Louisville KY 40203-2205
E-mail: Entechky@bellsouth.net
Website: www.councilonmr.org/enTECH.htm

(800) 890-1840, in state
(502) 574-1637
(502) 582-2448, fax

Western Kentucky Assistive Technology Consortium (WKATC)
Weaks Community Center
607 Poplar St.
PO Box 266
Murray KY 42071
E-mail: wkatc@wk.net

(270) 759-4233
(270) 759-4208, fax

Maryland

Learning Independence Through Computers, Inc. (LINC)
1001 Eastern Ave., 3rd Fl.
Baltimore MD 21202
E-mail: info@linc.org
Website: www.linc.org

(410) 659-5462
(410) 843-0219, TTY
(410) 659-5472, fax

Michigan

Michigan's Assistive Technology Resource (MATR)
1023 S. US 27, Suite B31
St. Johns MI 48879-2424
E-mail: matr@match.org
Website: www.cenmi.org/matr

(800) 274-7426
(989) 224-0333
(989) 224-0246, TTY
(989) 224-0330, fax

Minnesota

Simon Technology Center PACER Center
8161 Normandale Blvd.
Minnesota MN 55437-1044
E-mail: pacer@pacer.org
Website: www.pacer.org

(952) 838-9000
(952) 838-0190, TTY
(952) 838-0199, fax

Montana

Parents, Let's Unite for Kids (PLUK)
516 N. 32nd St.
Billings MT 59101
E-mail: plukinfo@pluk.org
Website: www.pluk.org

(800) 222-7585, in state
(406) 255-0540, voice, TTY
(406) 255-0523, fax

291

Alliance for
Technology
Access
Resource
Centers

New Jersey

Center for Assistive Tech & Inclusive Ed Studies (CATIES)
The College of New Jersey
PO Box 7718
Ewing NJ 08628-0718
E-mail: caties@tcnj.edu
Website: www.caties.tcnj.edu

(609) 771-3016
(609) 771-2995, TTY
(609) 637-5172, fax

TECHConnection—Assistive Technology Solutions
c/o Family Resource Associates, Inc.
35 Haddon Ave.
Shrewsbury NJ 07702
E-mail: tecconn@aol.com
Website: www.techconnection.org

(732) 747-5310
(732) 747-1896, fax

New York

Techspress/Resource Center for Independent Living
401–409 Columbia St.
PO Box 210
Utica NY 13503-0210
E-mail: tamara.mariotti@rcil.com
Website: www.rcil.com

(315) 797-4642
(315) 797-5837, TTY
(315) 797-4747, fax

North Carolina

Carolina Computer Access Center
401 East Ninth St.
Charlotte NC 28202
E-mail: ccacnc@bellsouth.com
Website: http://ccac.ataccess.org

(704) 342-3004
(704) 342-1513, fax

Ohio

Easter Seals Technology Resource Center
E-mail: k.leonard@goodwilldayton.org
Website: www.trcd.org

292

Computer
Resources
for People
with
Disabilities

Rhode Island

TechACCESS Center of Rhode Island
110 Jefferson Blvd., Suite 1
Warwick RI 02888-3854
E-mail: techaccess@techaccess-ri.org
Website: www.techaccess-ri.org

(800) 916-TECH, in state
(401) 463-0202, voice, TTY
(401) 463-3433, fax

Tennessee

East Tennessee Technology Access Center (ETTAC)
4918 North Broadway
Knoxville TN 37918
E-mail: etstactn@aol.com
Website: www.korrnet.org/ettac/

(865) 219-0130, voice, TTY
(865) 219-0137, fax

Mid-South Access Center for Technology
University of Memphis
Room 119, Patterson Hall
Memphis TN 38152
E-mail: act@memphis.edu
Website: www.coe.memphis.edu/ACT

(901) 678-1489
(901) 678-1318, TTY
(901) 678-3215, fax

Signal Center's Assistive Technology Center
109 North Germantown Rd.
Chattanooga TN 37411
E-mail: info@signal.chattanooga.net
Website: www.signalcenters.com

(423) 698-8528, ext. 242
(423) 698-3105, fax

Technology Access Center of Middle Tennessee
2222 Metrocenter Blvd., Suite 126
Nashville TN 37228
E-mail: techaccess@mindstate.com
Website: http://tac.ataccess.org

(800) 368-4651
(615) 248-6733, voice, TTY
(615) 259-2536, fax

West Tennessee Special Technology Access Resource Center (The STAR Center)
60 Lynoak Cove
Jackson TN 38305
E-mail: infostar@starcenter.tn.org
Website: www.starcenter.tn.org

(731) 668-3888
(731) 668-9664, TTY
(731) 668-1666, fax

Utah

The Computer Center for Citizens with Disabilities
The Utah Center for Assistive Technology

(888) 866-5550

1595 West 500 South (801) 887-9533, voice, TTY
Salt Lake City UT 84104 (801) 887-9382, fax
E-mail: cboogaar@utah.gov
Website: www.usor.state.ut.us/ucat/computers.htm

Virgin Islands

Virgin Islands Resource Center for the Disabled, Inc.
PO Box 308427 (340) 777-2253, voice, TTY
St. Thomas USVI 00803-8427 (340) 774-9330, fax
Website: www.vircd.org

Virginia

Tidewater Center for Technology Access (TCTA)
1413 Laskin Rd. (757) 474-6542, voice, TTY
Virginia Beach VA 23451 (757) 437-6540, fax
E-mail: tcta@aol.com
Website: http://tcta.ataccess.org

Assistive Technology Act

The Assistive Technology Act (formerly the Technology-Related Assistance for Individuals with Disabilities Act) provides funding to states to assist them in addressing the assistive-technology needs of individuals with disabilities. Programs vary widely from state to state. Contact your state project for specific information. A complete list of state projects, with contact information, can be obtained from RESNA's Technical Assistance Project at (703) 524-6686, extension 313, or found on RESNA's website at:

www.resna.org/taproject/at/statecontacts.html

Americans with Disabilities Act (ADA)

ADA Technology Resources

Many agencies and organizations provide support for the implementation of the Americans with Disabilities Act. The following agencies and organizations can provide you with information and referrals.

American Printing House for the Blind
PO Box 6085 (800) 223-1839 (U.S. and Canada)
1839 Frankfort Ave. (502) 895-2405

294

Computer
Resources
for People
with
Disabilities

Louisville KY 40206-0085   (502) 899-2274, fax
E-mail: info@aph.org
Website: www.aph.org

Job Accommodation Network (JAN)

A service of the Office of Disability Employment Policy (formerly President's Committee on Employment of People with Disabilities).

PO Box 6080   (800) 526-7234, voice, TTY (in U.S.)
Morgantown WV 26506-6080   (800) ADA-WORK (232-9675), voice, TTY
E-mail: jan@jan.wvu.edu   (304) 293-7186, voice, TTY (worldwide)
Website: www.jan.wvu.edu   (304) 293-5407, fax

Office of the Americans with Disabilities Act

U.S. Department of Justice   (800) 514-0301
Civil Rights Division   (202) 514-0301
Disabilities Rights Section NYAV   (800) 514-0383, TTY
950 Pennsylvania Ave. NW   (202) 514-0380, TTY
PO Box 66118   (202) 307-1198, fax
Washington DC 20530
Website: www.ada.gov

Equal Employment Opportunity Commission

1801 L St. NW   (800) 669-4000
Washington DC 20507   (202) 663-4900
Website: www.eeoc.gov   (800) 669-6820, TTY
  (202) 663-4494, TTY

ADA Technical-Assistance Programs

The National Institute on Disability and Rehabilitation Research (NIDRR) sponsors 10 federally funded agencies, called Disability and Business Technical Assistance Centers (DBTACs). There is one in each region of the country, and their purpose is to provide information and technical assistance on the ADA and on accessible information technology. Call (800) 949-4232, and your call will be directed to the assistance center for your region. (Spanish translation is also available at that number.) Or find your state in one of the regions listed below.

Region I: CT, ME, MA, NH, RI, VT

New England ADA and Accessible IT Center
Adaptive Environments Center, Inc.   (800) 949-4232, voice, TTY
374 Congress St., Suite 301   (617) 695-1225, voice, TTY
Boston MA 02210   (617) 695-0085, voice, TTY
E-mail: adainfo@newenglandada.org   (617) 482-8099, fax
Website: www.newenglandada.org

Region II: NJ, NY, PR

Northeast DBTAC Cerebral Palsy of New Jersey
354 South Broad St.   (609) 392-4004
Trenton NJ 08608   (609) 392-7044, TTY
E-mail: dbtac@cpofnj.org   (609) 392-3505, fax
Website: www.cpofnj.org

Region III: DE, DC, MD, PA, VA, WV

ADA and IT Information Center for the Mid-Atlantic Region
TransCen, Inc.   (800) 949-4232, voice, TTY
451 Hungerford Dr., Suite 607   (301) 217-0124, voice, TTY
Rockville MD 20850   (301) 217-0754, fax
E-mail: adainfo@transcen.org
Website: www.adainfo.org

Region IV: AL, FL, GA, KY, MS, NC, SC, TN

Georgia Center for Assistive Technology & Environmental Access (CATEA)
Southeast DBTAC
490 Tenth St.   (800) 949-4232, voice, TTY
Atlanta GA 30318   (404) 385-0636, voice, TTY
E-mail: sedbtacproject@catea.org   (404) 385-0641, fax
Website: www.sedbtac.org

Region V: IL, IN, MI, MN, OH, WI Great Lakes

ADA and IT Center (GLDBTAC)
West Roosevelt Rd., Room 405   (800) 949-4232, voice, TTY
Chicago IL 60608   (312) 413-1407, voice, TTY
E-mail: gldbtac@uic.edu   (312) 413-1856, fax
Website: www.adagreatlakes.org

Region VI: AR, LA, NM, OK, TX

Disability Law Resource Project (DLRP)
Independent Living Research Utilization (ILRU)   (800) 949-3944
South Shepherd Blvd., Suite 1000   (713) 520-0232, voice
Houston TX 77019   (713) 520-5136, TTY
E-mail: ilru@ilru.org *or* dlrp@ilru.org   (713) 520-5785, fax
Website: www.ilru.org *or* www.dlrp.org

Region VII: IA, KS, NB, MO

The Great Plains ADA & IT Center
100 Corporate Lake Dr.   (800) 949-4232, voice, TTY
Columbia MO 65203   (573) 882-3600, voice, TTY
E-mail: ada@missouri.edu   (573) 884-4925, fax
Website: www.adaproject.org

296

Computer
Resources
for People
with
Disabilities

Region VIII: CO, MT, ND, SD, UT, WY
Rocky Mountain DBTAC ADA/IT Center
Meeting the Challenge, Inc.   (800) 949-4232, voice, TTY
3630 Sinton Rd., Suite 103   (719) 444-0268, voice, TTY
Colorado Springs CO 80907   (719) 444-0269, fax
E-mail: rmdbtac@mtc-inc.com
Website: www.adainformation.org

Region IX: AZ, CA, HI, NV, PB
Pacific ADA & IT Center (Pacific DBTAC)
555 12th St., Suite 1030   (510) 285-5600, voice, TTY
Oakland CA 94607-4040   (510) 285-5614, fax
E-mail: adatech@pdbtac.com
Website: www.pacdbtac.org

Region X: AK, ID, OR, WA
Northwest ADA & IT Center
Oregon Health Sciences University   (800) 949-4232, voice, TTY
PO Box 574   (503) 494-4001, voice, TTY
Portland OR 97207-0574   (503) 418-0785, fax
E-mail: nwada@ohsu.edu
Website: www.nwada.org

Organizations

There are thousands of organizations that serve people with disabilities. The
ones listed here represent some of the many national organizations (as well
as the U.S. offices of international organizations) that have an interest in technology for disabled people and that can provide technology-related services,
information, or referrals.

AAC Institute
338 Meadville St.   (330) 464-7877
Edinboro PA 16412
E-mail: bromich@aacinstitute.org
Website: www.aacinstitute.org

Alexander Graham Bell Association for the Deaf
3417 Volta Pl. NW   (202) 337-5220, voice, TTY
Washington DC 20007-2778   (202) 337-8314, fax
Website: www.agbell.org

Alliance for Public Technology
919 18th St. NW, Suite 900   (202) 263-2970, voice, TTY

Washington DC 20006   (202) 263-2960, fax
E-mail: apt@apt.org
Website: www.apt.org

Alliance for Technology Access
1304 Southpoint Blvd., Suite 240   (707) 778-3011
Petaluma CA 94954   (707) 778-3015, TTY
E-mail: ATAinfo@ATAccess.org   (707) 765-2080, fax
Website: www.ATAccess.org

American Foundation for the Blind
National Technology Center   (800) 232-5463
11 Penn Plaza, Suite 300   (212) 502-7642
New York NY 10001   (212) 502-7773, fax
E-mail: afbinfo@afb.net
Website: www.afb.org

American Occupational Therapy Association (AOTA)
PO Box 31220   (301) 652-2682
4720 Montgomery Ln.   (800) 377-8555, TTY
Bethesda MD 20824-1220   (301) 652-7711, fax
E-mail: praota@aota.org
Website: www.aota.org

American Printing House for the Blind
1839 Frankfort Ave.   (800) 223-1839
PO Box 6085   (502) 895-2405
Louisville KY 40206-0085   (502) 899-2274, fax
E-mail: info@aph.org
Website: www.aph.org

American Speech-Language-Hearing Association (ASHA)
10801 Rockville Pike   (800) 638-8255, voice, TTY
Rockville MD 20852   (301) 897-5700, members
E-mail: actioncenter@asha.org   (301) 897-0157, TTY
Website: www.asha.org   (301) 571-0457, fax

The Arc (formerly Association for Retarded Citizens)
The Arc of the United States   (301) 565-3842
1010 Wayne Ave., Suite 650   (301) 565-3843, fax
Silver Spring MD 20910   (301) 565-5342, fax
E-mail: info@thearc.org
Website: http://thearc.org

Association of University Centers on Disabilities
8630 Fenton St., Suite 410   (301) 588-8252

298

Computer
Resources
for People
with
Disabilities

Silver Spring MD 20910   (301) 588-2842, fax
E-mail: kmusheno@aucd.org
Website: www.aucd.org

Autism Society of America
7910 Woodmont Ave., Suite 300   (800) 3-AUTISM (328-8476)
Bethesda MD 20814-3015   (301) 657-0881
E-mail: info@autism-society.org   (301) 657-0869, fax
Website: www.autism-society.org

Center for Applied Special Technology (CAST)
40 Harvard Mills Sq., Suite 3   (781) 245-2212
Wakefield MA 01880-3233   (781) 245-5212, fax
E-mail: cast@cast.org   (781) 245-9320, TTY
Website: www.cast.org

Center for Assistive Technology & Environmental Access
Georgia Institute of Technology   (404) 894-4960, voice, TTY
490 10th St., NW   (404) 894-9320, fax
Atlanta GA 30332-0156
Website: www.catea.org

Center for Best Practices in Early Childhood Education
Western Illinois University   (309) 298-1634
27 Horrabin Hall   (309) 298-2305, fax
Macomb IL 61455-1390
Website: www.wiu.edu/users/mimacp/wiu/

Center for Information Technology Accommodation
GSA 18th and F St. NW, Room 1234   (202) 501-4906
MC:MWA   (202) 501-6269, fax
Washington DC 20405
E-mail: quentis.scott@gsa.gov
Website: www.gsa.gov

Community Technology Centers' Network (CTCNet)
1436 U St. NW, Suite 104   (202) 462-1200
Washington DC 20009   (202) 462-3892
E-mail: info@ctcnet.org
Website: www.ctcnet.org

The Council for Exceptional Children (CEC)
1110 North Glebe Rd., Suite 300   (703) 620-3660
Arlington VA 22201   (703) 264-9446, TTY
E-mail: service@cec.sped.org   (703) 264-9494, fax
Website: www.cec.sped.org

Independent-Living Centers

For a directory of sites in your state, contact: (713) 520-0232
ILRU (713) 520-5136, TTY
2323 South Shepherd, Suite 1000 (713) 520-5785, fax
Houston TX 77019
E-mail: ilru@ilru.org
Website: www.ilru.org

Infinitec

UCP Chicago (312) 368-0380
160 N. Wacker Dr. (312) 368-0179, TTY
Chicago IL 60606 (312) 368-0018, fax
Website: www.infinitec.org

International Braille and Technology Center for the Blind

National Federation for the Blind (410) 659-9314
1800 Johnson St., Suite 300 (410) 685-5653, fax
Baltimore MD 21230-4998
E-mail: nfb@nfb.org
Website: www.nfb.org

International Dyslexia Society (formerly the Orton Dyslexia Society)

Chester Building, Suite 382 (800) 331-0688
8600 La Salle Rd. (410) 296-0232
Baltimore MD 21286-2044 (410) 321-5069, fax
E-mail: info@interdys.org
Website: www.interdys.org

International Society for Augmentative and Alternative Communication (ISAAC)

49 The Donway West, Suite 308 (416) 385-0351
Toronto ON M3C 3M9 (416) 385-0352, fax
Canada
E-mail: secretariat@isaac-online.org
Website: www.isaac-online.org

International Society for Technology and Education

1710 Rhode Island Ave. NW, Suite 900 (202) 861-7777
Washington DC 20036 (202) 861-0888
E-mail: iste@iste.org
Website: www.iste.org

Job Accommodation Network (JAN)

West Virginia University (800) 526-7234 voice, TTY
PO Box 6080 (800) ADA-WORK (232-9675), voice, TTY

300

Computer
Resources
for People
with
Disabilities

Morgantown WV 26506   (304) 293-7186 voice, TTY (worldwide)
E-mail: jan@jan.wvu.edu
Website: http://janweb.icdi.wvu.edu

Learning Disabilities Association of America
4156 Library Rd.   (412) 341-1515
Pittsburgh PA 15234   (412) 344-0224, fax
E-mail: info@ldaamerica.org
Website: www.ldanatl.org

National Association of Protection and Advocacy Systems, Inc.
900 Second St. NE, Suite 211   (202) 408-9514
Washington DC 20002   (202) 408-9520, TTY, fax
E-mail: napas@earthlink.net
Website: www.protectionandadvocacy.com

National Center for Disability Services
201 I.U. Willets Rd.   (516) 465-1400
Albertson NY 11507
Website: www.ncds.org

National Center for Learning Disabilities
381 Park Ave. South, Suite 1401   (888) 575-7373
New York NY 10016   (212) 545-7510
Website: www.ncld.org   (212) 545-9665, fax

Laurent Clerc National Deaf Education Center
Gallaudet University   (202) 651-5051
800 Florida Ave. NE   (202) 651-5000, voice, TTY
Washington DC 20002-3695
E-mail: iscs.clerccenter@gallaudet.edu
Website: http://clerccenter.gallaudet.edu

Lighthouse International
New York City Headquarters   (800) 829-0500
111 E. 59th St.   (212) 821-9200
New York NY 10022-1202   (212) 821-9713, TTY
Website: www.lighthouse.org   (212) 821-9707, fax

National Dissemination Center for Children with Disabilities (NICHCY)
PO Box 1492   (800) 695-0285, voice, TTY
Washington DC 20013-1492   (202) 884-8200, voice, TTY
E-mail: nichcy@aed.org   (202) 884-8441, fax
Website: www.nichcy.org

National Easter Seal Society

230 West Monroe St., Suite 1800
Chicago IL 60606-4802
E-mail: nessinfo@seals.com
Website: www.easter-seals.org

(800) 221-6827
(312) 726-6200
(312) 726-4258, TTY
(312) 726-1494, fax

National Lekotek Center

2100 Ridge Ave.
Evanston IL 60201-2796
E-mail: lekotek@lekotek.org
Website: www.lekotek.org

(800) 366-PLAY (366-7529)
(847) 328-0001, voice, TTY
(847) 328-5514, fax

National Rehabilitation Information Center (NARIC)

1010 Wayne Ave., Suite 800
Silver Spring MD 20910-5633
E-mail: naricinfo@kra.com
Website: www.naric.com

(800) 346-2742
(301) 562-2401, fax

National Technical Institute for the Deaf

Rochester Institute of Technology
One Lomb Memorial Dr.
Rochester NY 14623-5604
E-mail: NTIDMC@rit.edu
Website: http://ntidweb.rit.edu

(716) 475-2411
(716) 475-2810, TTY
(716) 475-6500, fax

Office of Disability Employment Policy (formerly President's Committee on Employment of People with Disabilities)

U.S. Dept. of Labor
200 Constitution Ave. NW
Washington DC 20210
Website: www.dol.gov/odep

(202) 376-6200

Parent Training and Information Centers

To find the PTI in your state, contact:
Technical Assistance Alliance for Parent Centers
PACER Center
8161 Normandale Blvd.
Minneapolis MN 55437-1044
E-mail: alliance@taalliance.org
Website: www.taalliance.org

(888) 248-0822 (in state)
(952) 838-9000
(952) 838-0190, TTY
(952) 838-0199, fax

Recording for the Blind and Dyslexic

20 Roszel Rd.
Princeton NJ 08540
E-mail: info@rfbd.org
Website: www.rfbd.org

(800) 803-7201, customer service
(609) 452-0606
(609) 987-8116, fax

302

Computer
Resources
for People
with
Disabilities

Rehabilitation International
25 East 21 St.
New York NY 10010
E-mail: rehabintl@rehab-international.org
Website: www.rehab-international.org

(212) 420-1500
(212) 505-0871, fax

Rehabilitation Engineering and Assistive Technology Society of North America (RESNA)
1700 N. Moore St., Suite 1540
Arlington VA 22209-1903
E-mail: info@resna.org
Website: www.resna.org

(703) 524-6686
(703) 524-6639, TTY
(703) 524-6630, fax

SeniorNet
121 Second St., 7th Fl.
San Francisco CA 94105
Website: www.seniornet.org

(415) 495-4990
(415) 495-3999, fax

Sensory Access Foundation
1142 West Evelyn Ave.
Sunnyvale CA 94086
E-mail: receptionist@sensoryaccess.com
Website: www.sensoryaccess.com

(408) 245-7330
(408) 245-3762, fax

TASH (Association for Persons with Severe Handicaps)
29 West Susquehanna, Suite 210
Baltimore MD 21204
Website: www.tash.org

(410) 828-8274
(410) 828-1306, TTY
(410) 828-6706, fax

Technology and Media (TAM)
The Council for Exceptional Children
1110 North Glebe Rd., Suite 300
Arlington VA 22201-5704
Website: www.tamcec.org

(888) CEC-SPED (232-7733)
(703) 620-3660
(703) 264-9446, TTY
(703) 264-9494, fax

Telecommunications for the Deaf Incorporated (TDI)
8630 Fenton St., Suite 604
Silver Spring MD 20910-3803
E-mail: info@tdi-online.org
Website: www.tdi-online.org

(301) 589-3786
(301) 589-3006, TTY
(301) 589-3797, fax

Through the Looking Glass
2198 Sixth St., Suite 100
Berkeley CA 94710-2204
E-mail: TLG@lookingglass.org
Website: www.lookingglass.org

(800) 644-2666
(510) 848-1112
(800) 804-1616, TTY
(510) 848-4445, fax

Trace Research and Development Center

University of Wisconsin-Madison
2107 Engineering Centers Bldg.
1550 Engineering Dr.
Madison WI 53706
E-mail: info@trace.wisc.edu
Website: http://trace.wisc.edu

(608) 262-6966
(608) 263-5408, TTY
(608) 262-8848, fax

United Cerebral Palsy Associations

1660 L St. NW, Suite 700
Washington DC 20036
E-mail: ucpnatl@ucpa.org
Website: www.ucpa.org

(800) USA-5UCP (872-5827)
(800) 872-5827, voice, TTY
(202) 776-0406
(202) 776-0414, fax

United Nations Persons with Disabilities Website

Focal Point on Disability
Division for Social Policy and Development
Department of Economic and Social Affairs
United Nations Secretariat
Two United Nations Plaza, DC2-1372
New York NY 10017
Website: www.un.org/esa/socdev/enable/

(212) 963-0111, fax

United States Society for Augmentative and Alternative Communication (USSAAC)

Duke University Medical Center
Box 3888
Durham NC 27710
E-mail: aac-rerc@mc.duke.edu
Website: www.aac-rerc.org

(919) 681-9983
(919) 681-9984, fax

International Resources

The international assistive-technology and disability resources included here represent a starting point for finding information around the globe. For more specific locations, try contacting an organization within the region you are interested in and ask for a referral.

Abledata

A comprehensive list of international assistive-technology sites.
www.abledata.com/text2/internat.htm

304

Computer
Resources
for People
with
Disabilities

Inclusion International
E-mail: info@inclusion-international.org
Website: www.inclusion-international.org

Africa

Disabled People's International: Regional Development Offices, Africa Region
Mohamed Fall +223-673-1063
P.O. Box 2609 +223-673-1079
Bamako - West Africa +223-220-0474, fax
Mali
E-mail: dpiafrica_rdobamako@hotmail.com *or* mohamedfall@hotmail.com
Website: www.dpi.org/en/locations/regions/regions.htm

Asia

Disabled People's International: Regional Development Offices, Asia/Pacific Region
Topong Kulkhanchit +662-503-4446
325 Bonstreet Rd.
Muangthong Thani Bangpood
Pakkred, Nonthaburi 11120
Thailand
E-mail: handipro@loxinfo.co.th

Disabled People's Association, Singapore
150A, Pandan Gardens, #02-00 +65-6899-1220
Day Care Center (Ayer Rajah Community Center) +65-6899-1232, fax
Singapore 609342
E-mail: dpa@dpa.org.sg
Website: www.dpa.org.sg

Information Resources for People with Disabilities, Japan
E-mail: sensui@sd.soft.iwate-pu.ac.jp
Website: www.sd.soft.iwate-pu.ac.jp/sensui/index-e.html (in English and Japanese)

Japan Council on Independent-Living Centers
Shimamula Building 102 +042-529-1169
Tachikawa-shi nishiki-cho 1-3-13, Tokyo, Japan +042-525-4757, fax
E-mail: asv69068@pcvan.or.jp *or* jil@d1.dion.ne.jp
Website: www.d1.dion.ne.jp/~jil/ (in Japanese)

Australia

Australian Rehabilitation & Assistive Technology Association (ARATA)
PO Box 278
Glenorie NSW 2157
Australia
E-mail: tonyharman@bigfoot.com
Website: www.e-bility.com/arata/index.php

Disability Information Resource Center, Inc.
195 Gilles St.   +08-8236-0555
Adelaide SA 5000   +08-8236-0566, fax
Australia   +08-8223-7579, TTY
E-mail: dirc@dircsa.org.au
Website: www.dircsa.org.au
Website: www.enable.net.au

Central America/South America

**Disabled People's International: Regional Development Offices,
Asia/Pacific Region**
Federación Nacional de Discapacitados Dominicanos (FENADID)
Teófilo Alarcón   +809-582-2396
Calle 6 No. 11, La Zurza   +809-697-0319, cell
Santiago de los Caballeros   +809-582-2396, fax
Dominican Republic
E-mail: fenadid@hotmail.com
Website: www.dpi.org/en/locations/regions/regions.htm

Europe

**Association for the Advancement of Assistive Technology in Europe
(AAATE)**
AAATE c/o Danish Centre   +45-43-52-70-72, fax
Gregersensvej
DK-2630 Taastrup
Denmark
E-mail: AAATE@hmi.dk
Website: http://139.91.151.134/

The Danish Centre for Technical Aids for Rehabilitation and Education
Danish Centre   +45-43-99-33-22
Gregersensvej   +45-43-52-70-72, fax
DK-2630 Taastrup

306

Computer
Resources
for People
with
Disabilities

Denmark
E-mail: hmi@hmi.dk
Website: www.hmi.dk/

European Design for All: E-Accessibility Network (EDeAN)

Danish Centre   +45-87-41-24-38
Gregersensvej 38   +45-86-75-36-67, fax
Dk-2630 Taastrup
Denmark
E-mail: edean@hmi.dk
Website: www.e-accessibility.org

Forschungsinstitut Technologie-Behindertenhilfe (FTB)

Grundschötteler Straße 40   +49-0-2335-9681-0
D-58300 Wetter/Ruhr   +49-0-2335-9681-19, fax
Deutschland
E-mail: webmaster@ftb-volmarstein.de
Website: http://en.ftb-net.de (in English)

Hacavie

E-mail: demande@hacavie.com
Website: www.hacavie.com (in French)

Servizio Informazioni e Valutazione Ausili (SIVA)

SIVA   +39-02-40308340
via Capecelatro 66, I-20148
Milano
Italy
E-mail: ausili@siva.it
Website: www.siva.it (in Italian and English)

Swiss Foundation for Rehabilitation Technology

Charmettes 10b   +41-32/732-97-77
Case postale   +41-32/730-58-63, fax
CH-2006 Neuchâtel
Switzerland
E-mail: info@fst.ch
Website: www.fst.ch/ (in French and German; partially in Italian and English)

World Federation of the Deaf

PO Box 65   +358-9-580-3573, TTY
00401 Helsinki   +358-9-580-3572, fax
Finland
E-mail: info@wfdnews.org

Council of Canadians with Disabilities

32 Chemin Croissant (819) 459-2243
Chelsea, Québec J9B 2J8 (819) 459-3665, fax
Canada
E-mail: estey@sympatico.ca
Website: www.dpi.org/en/locations/regions/regions.htm

Council of Canadians with Disabilities

Somerset Building, 926-294 Portage Ave. (204) 947-0303
Winnipeg, Manitoba, R3C 0B9 (204) 942-4625, fax
Canada
E-mail: ccd@pcs.mb.ca
Website: www.dpi.org/en/locations/regions/regions.htm

International Society for Augmentative and Alternative Communication (ISAAC)

49 The Donway West, Suite 308 (416) 385-0351
Toronto ON M3C 3M9 (416) 385-0352
Canada
E-mail: secretariat@isaac-online.org
Website: www.isaac-online.org (in English)

Conferences and Other Events

The conferences listed below are key annual events that address technology and people with disabilities. This list is not exhaustive. Literally hundreds of conferences take place each year that relate to this field. You can find out about numerous state, regional, and local conferences by contacting your community technology resources and the Assistive Technology Act (Tech Act) project in your state.

Abilities Expo

Corporate Office (617) 267-6500
Advanstar, Inc. (617) 267-6900
545 Boylston St.
Boston MA 02116
E-mail: info@advanstar.com
Website: www.abilitiesexpo.com

308

Computer
Resources
for People
with
Disabilities

Alliance for Public Technology/Policy Forum
919 18th St. NW, Suite 900   (202) 263-2970, voice, TTY
Washington DC 20006   (202) 263-2960, fax
E-mail: apt@apt.org
Website: www.apt.org

American Speech-Language-Hearing Association (ASHA) Convention
10801 Rockville Pike   (800) 638-8255
Rockville MD 20852
E-mail: webmaster@asha.org
Website: www.asha.org

American Occupational Therapy Association (AOTA) Annual Conference & Exposition
4720 Montgomery Ln.   (301) 652-2682
PO Box 31220   (800) 377-8555, TTY
Bethesda MD 20824   (301) 652-7711, fax
Website: www.aota.org

Assistive Technology Industry Association Conference & Exhibition
401 North Michigan Ave.   (877) 687-2842
Chicago IL 60611   (312) 494-3015, fax
E-mail: info@ATIA.org
Website: www.ATIA.org

CAMA (Communication Aid Manufacturers Association) Workshops
PO Box 1039   (800) 441-CAMA (441-2262)
Evanston IL 60204-1039
E-mail: cama@northshore.net
Website: www.aacproducts.org

Closing the Gap Annual Conference
PO Box 68   (507) 248-3294
Henderson MN 56044   (507) 248-3810, fax
Website: www.closingthegap.com

International Society for Augmentative and Alternative Communication (ISAAC) Biennial Conference
49 The Donway West, Suite 308   (416) 385-0351
Toronto ON M3C 3M9   (416) 385-0352, fax
Canada
E-mail: secretariat@isaac-online.org
Website: www.isaac-online.org

Learning Disabilities Association of America International Conference

4156 Library Rd.   (412) 341-1515
Pittsburgh PA 15234   (412) 344-0224, fax
E-mail: info@ldaamerica.org
Website: www.ldanatl.org

RESNA International Conference

1700 N. Moore St., Suite 1540   (703) 524-6686
Arlington VA 22209-1903   (703) 524-6639, TTY
E-mail: info@resna.org   (703) 524-6630, fax
Website: www.resna.org

Technology and Media (TAM)

The Council for Exceptional Children   (888) CEC-SPED (232-7733)
1110 North Glebe Rd., Suite 300   (703) 620-3660
Arlington VA 22201-5704   (866) 915-5000, TTY only
Website: www.cec.sped.org   (703) 264-9494, fax

Technology and Persons with Disabilities Annual Conference

California State University, Northridge (CSUN)(818) 885-2578, voice, TTY
Center on Disabilities   (818) 677-4929, fax
18111 Nordoff St.
Northridge CA 91330-8340
E-mail: ctrdis@csun.edu
Website: www.csun.edu/cod/

Technology, Reading & Learning Difficulties International Conference

Educational Computer Conferences, Inc.   (888) 594-1249
19 Calvert Ct.   (510) 594-1249
Piedmont CA 94611   (510) 594-1838, fax
E-mail: info@trld.com
Website: www.trld.com

Publications

The following list, which is intended to be illustrative rather than exhaustive, includes several types of publications that focus on or regularly cover assistive technology. Some publications are available only through the Internet. Some print-only publications may be available at your local public or college library.

310

Computer
Resources
for People
with
Disabilities

Newsletters, Magazines, and Journals

AccessWorld: Technology for Consumers with Visual Impairments
American Foundation for the Blind
Bimonthly; free online starting January 2004; available in multiple electronic formats
Website: www.afb.org/accessworld.asp

Alternatively Speaking
Augmentative Communication, Inc.   (831) 649-3050
One Surf Way, #237   (831) 646-5428, fax
Monterey CA 93940
Available in print only; published three times annually
Website: www.augcominc.com

Assistive Technology for People with Disabilities
TECH-NJ, The College of New Jersey
Annual; available free online (HTML) or in print by request
Website: www.tcnj.edu/~technj/

Assistive Technology Journal
RESNA   (703) 524-6686, ext. 306
1700 N. Moore St., Suite 1540   (703) 524-6639, TTY
Arlington VA 22209
Published semiannually; available in print
E-mail: journal@resna.org
Website:
www.resna.org/ProfResources/Publications/ATJournal/Subscribe.php

AT Journal
AT Network/California Assistive Technology Systems
Monthly; free online (HTML)
Website: www.atnet.org/news/

Augmentative and Alternative Communication
ISAAC
Taylor & Francis
Published quarterly; available online
Website: www.tandf.co.uk/journals/subscription.html

Augmentative Communication News
Augmentative Communication, Inc.
Available in print only
Website: http://shop.augcominc.com/osb/showitem.cfm/Category/38

Braille Monitor

National Federation of the Blind (410) 659-9314
1800 Johnson St.
Baltimore MD 21230
Monthly; free online (HTML or text file) or via e-mail; also available in print, Braille, or cassette
Website: www.nfb.org/bralmons.htm

The Catalyst

Western Center for Microcomputers in Special Education, Inc.
1259 El Camino Real, #275 (650) 855-8064
Menlo Park CA 94025
Available in print; selected articles available free online (PDF)
Website: www.thecatalyst.us/index.html

Closing the Gap

526 Main St. (507) 248-3294
PO Box 68
Henderson MN 56044
Bimonthly; newsletter and resource directory available in print version or online
Website: www.closingthegap.com/ctg2/subscribe/indexSub.lasso

CONNSense Bulletin

Available free online (HTML)
Website: www.connsensebulletin.com

Deaf Today

Daily; free online (HTML)
Website: www.deaftoday.com/news

Disability World

IDEAS Project
4–6 issues per year; free online; available in multiple formats in English and Spanish
www.disabilityworld.org

E-Letter

Center for an Accessible Society
Weekly; free via e-mail; archive free online (HTML)
Website: www.accessiblesociety.org

Exceptional Parent Magazine

65 East Route 4 (201) 489-4111
River Edge NJ 07661

312

Computer
Resources
for People
with
Disabilities

Published 10 times annually; includes an annual resource guide; some articles available online
Website: www.eparent.com

Journal of Special Education Technology

Council for Exceptional Children	(888) CEC-SPED (232-7733)
1110 North Glebe Rd., Suite 300	(703) 620-3663
Arlington VA 22201-5704	(703) 264-9446, TTY

Quarterly; available free online (HTML) or in a print version for $40/year
Website: http://jset.unlv.edu/shared/volsmenu.html

Public Tech Notes

Alliance for Public Technology
Monthly; free online (HTML, PDF)
Website: http://apt.org/publictech/

RehabWire

National Rehabilitation Information Center (NARIC)
Average of 10 issues/year; free online (HTML, PDF)
Website: www.naric.com/RehabWire

Special Education Technology Practice

c/o Knowledge by Design, Inc.	(414) 962-0120
5907 N. Kent Ave.	
Whitefish Bay WI 53217	

Published bimonthly; available in print only
Website: www.setp.net

Volta Voices

Alexander Graham Bell Association for the Deaf and Hard of Hearing	
3417 Volta Pl. NW	(202) 337-5220
Washington DC 20007	(202) 337-5221

Published bimonthly; available in print only
Website: www.agbell.org/periodicals.cfm

Books

To stay informed on **books in print related to disability and technology**, visit the following three websites:

www.ldresources.com

www.amazon.com

www.specialneeds.com

To locate books that are **out of print**, try www.abebooks.com.

Access Aware: Extending Your Reach to People with Disabilities. J. Kailes, R. Holland, M. Lester, and S. Brown. San Rafael, CA: Alliance for Technology Access, 2001.

Adapting PCs for Disabilities. J. Lazarro. Reading, MA: Addison-Wesley, 1996.

Adaptive Technologies for Learning and Work Environments (2nd edition). J. Lazzaro. Chicago: American Library Association Editions, 2001.

Adaptive Technology for the Internet. B. T. Mates. Chicago: American Library Association, 2000.

Assistive Technologies: Principles and Practice (2nd edition). A. M. Cook and S. M. Hussey. St. Louis, MO: Mosby, Inc., 2001.

Assistive Technology for People with Disabilities. D. P. Bryant and B. R. Bryant. Upper Saddle River, NJ: Pearson Allyn & Bacon, 2002.

Assistive Technology: Matching Device and Consumer for Successful Rehabilitation. M. J. Sherer, editor. Washington, DC: APA Books, 2002.

Assistive Technology Solutions for IEP Teams. S. L. Purcell and D. Grant. Verona, WI: Attainment Company, Inc. 2002.

Augmentative and Alternative Communication: Management of Severe Communication Disorders in Children and Adults (2nd edition). D. Beukelman and P. Mirenda. Baltimore: Paul H. Brookes Publishing, 1998.

Birth to Five: Early Childhood Special Education (2nd edition). F. Bowe. New York: Delmar, 1999.

Book of Possibilities: Activities Using Simple Technology (Elementary). H. Canfield. Minneapolis: AbleNet, 1998.

Book of Possibilities: Activities Using Simple Technology (Secondary). H. Canfield. Minneapolis: AbleNet, 1998.

Choosing Assistive Devices: A Guide for Users and Professionals. H. Pain, D. L. McLellan, S. Gore, and S. L. Kuman. London: Jessica Kingsley Pub., 2003.

The Complete Directory for People with Disabilities 2003: A Comprehensive Source Book for Individuals and Professionals (11th edition). L. Mars. Lakeville, CT: Grey House, 2002.

Connecting to Learn: Educational and Assistive Technology for People with Disabilities. M. J. Scherer. Washington, DC: APA Books, 2003.

314

Computer
Resources
for People
with
Disabilities

Early Communication Skills for Children with Down Syndrome: A Guide for Parents and Professionals (2nd edition). L. Kumin. Rockville, MD: Woodbine House, 2003.

Family Guide to Assistive Technology. K. Kelker, R. Holt, and J. Sullivan. Cambridge, MA: Brookline Books, 2001.

Financial Aid for the Disabled and Their Families, 2002–2004. Gail A. Schlachter and R. David Weber. El Dorado Hills, CA: Reference Service Press, 2003.

Living in a State of Stuck: How Assistive Technology Impacts the Lives of People with Disabilities (3rd edition). M. J. Scherer. Cambridge, MA: Brookline Books, 2000.

Mindstorms: Children, Computers, and Powerful Ideas (2nd edition). S. Papert. New York: Basic Books, 1999.

Reflections from a Unicorn. R. Creech. Greenville, NC: RC Publishing Company, 1992.

Special Educational Needs and the Internet: Issues for the Inclusive Classroom. C. Abbott, editor. New York: Routledge, 2002.

Special Education Technology: Classroom Applications. R. B. Lewis. Belmont, CA: Wadsworth Publishing, 1999.

Spinal Network: The Total Wheelchair Resource Book. B. Corbet and J. Dobbs, editors. Santa Monica, CA: Nine Lives Press, 2002.

Technology for Inclusion: Meeting the Special Needs of All Students (4th edition). M. Male. Boston: Allyn & Bacon, 2002.

Technology for Students with Disabilities: A Decision Maker's Resource Guide. A collaborative production of the National School Boards Association and the Office of Special Education Programs, Office of Special Education and Rehabilitative Service, U.S. Department of Education. 1997.

Total Augmentative Communication in the Early Childhood Classroom. L. J. Burkhart. Eldersburg, MD: Linda J. Burkhart, 1993.

Books for Librarians

Books of special interest to **librarians** about providing access for their patrons include:

Nothing about Me…Without Me: Involving People with Disabilities in Planning Public Library Services. R. J. Rubin. Sacramento, CA: California State Library, 2002.

Planning for Library Services for People with Disabilities: A Process for Libraries. R. J. Rubin. Chicago: ASCLA, 2001.

Preparing Staff to Serve Patrons with Disabilities: A How-To-Do-It Manual for Librarians. C. Deines and C. Van Fleet. New York: Neal-Schuman, 1995.

Internet Resources

The Internet is often described as a "network of networks." This means you can access information and resources from computers across the world as easily as you can from the computer on your desk. There are a variety of formats people typically use to get information. Among the most common is the World Wide Web.

The World Wide Web (www) offers extensive information and resources in a format that is comfortable and intuitive for many people. Reviewing this information requires software known as a browser. Some popular browsers include Netscape, Microsoft Internet Explorer, Mosaic, and Lynx, among many others. Browsers are graphics oriented, which creates potential barriers for users who rely on text-based material. Websites designed in accordance with the accessibility guidelines developed by the Web Accessibility Initiative (www.w3.org/WAI/) are accessible to all individuals, including those using text-based browsers and screen readers.

Each website has an address known as its URL (uniform resource locator). Typing in the URL allows you to visit the website you have indicated.

Using Search Engines

The best way to identify web pages and newsgroups and to gather information on the Internet is to use a search engine. A search engine compares keywords typed in by the user to information provided by the owner of the website about the content of the site. Meta search engines combine the results of several search engines and present them to the user. One such meta search engine is called Seti-search. Seti-search presents the information from both single and meta search engines in a format that can be used easily by people with a range of disabilities and by people who use assistive technology. The site even allows the user to change the display on the page and to save the settings for subsequent visits. The web address for Seti-search is www.seti-search.com.

Internet Resources for People with Disabilities

Internet services of specific interest to people with disabilities are increasing in number all the time. Many of the key commercial services offer resources

316

———

Computer
Resources
for People
with
Disabilities

for people with disabilities. Many organizations serving people with disabilities have developed their own web pages (or homepages), e-mail capacity, and electronic-bulletin-board systems. The number of World Wide Web sites and other Internet resources focused on disability is extensive and expanding. The lists change often, and so do online addresses, so the services and systems listed below are included to give you a sense of the scope of the field and where to begin exploring.

These services vary in cost, and the rates change frequently due to heavy competition, so it pays to comparison shop before signing up.

America Online

AOL offers a disABILITIES forum with a broad range of information, databases, chat rooms, software libraries, and presentations. You can get information on many topics of interest to people with disabilities, including the ADA, job accommodations, social security, and relevant organizations, to name a few. The site also offers opportunities for interactive sessions with others. AOL will send you its proprietary graphic-interface along with an introductory offer if you call customer service at (800) 827-6364. It is also possible to access the AOL website with a browser at www.aol.com. AOL has added features that make it friendlier to those using screen readers and other assistive technology. For further information, AOL has created a special section of its web page for information regarding accessibility: www.aol.com/accessibility.

Dimenet

Dimenet (Disabled Individuals' Movement for Equality Network) is an on-line service that provides access for communication and information sharing among individuals involved in the disability-rights and independent-living movements. The network is comprehensive and consumer controlled. Because it was designed with access in mind, it is easy to navigate. The phone numbers you must dial through your modem to reach Dimenet are: (508) 820-3376 in Framingham, Massachusetts; (937) 341-5205 in Dayton, Ohio; and (724) 223-6160 in Washington, Pennsylvania. If you live outside of these three cities, expect to pay long-distance charges. Once you are connected, the first thing you do is type "dime" in lowercase letters and press <ENTER>. To create an account, type "new" and press <ENTER>. Once you have signed on to Dimenet, you can "TELNET" from other systems by entering "Dimenet.org." For more information visit its website: www.dimenet.com.

SeniorNet

SeniorNet is an organization dedicated to building a community of computer-using seniors. It has over 10,000 members. SeniorNet operates 200 learning centers and hosts active discussion areas on its website. For more information, contact SeniorNet at (415) 495-4990; fax, (415) 495-3999. Postal address: 121 Second Street, 7th Floor, San Francisco CA 94105. Website: www.seniornet.org.

Using the Internet

Commercial services (such as AOL and others) provide an easy way to get onto the Internet. The advantages of using a commercial service include ease in getting started and low cost. Another advantage is the substantial amount of disability-related content available on most commercial services. Almost all of them now feature areas for disability-related software, resources, sharing, and support.

If you are planning to spend a significant amount of time on the Internet, however, you may want to consider using an Internet service provider (ISP). These companies provide direct, unlimited access to the Internet via local phone numbers for a monthly rate. In addition, a variety of options for high-speed connection are now available using broadband services such as DSL and cable. Check with companies in your area to see if these services are available. Although the monthly rates for high-speed connections are generally higher than they are for dial-up service, they offer faster, more stable connections to the Internet.

Yahoo, Hotmail, Net Zero, USA Datanet, and Juno represent options for low-cost or no-cost Internet and e-mail access. The access is generally free because you are exposed to advertising from the provider. Competition for Internet exposure will continue to rapidly change the options for Internet access.

Selecting an Internet Service Provider (ISP)

For people who use assistive technology, selecting an ISP is an important part of using your technology on the Internet. In general, companies that allow the end user to choose their browser and e-mail package are more compatible with assistive technology. Select your ISP based on its compatibility with products that optimize the effectiveness of the assistive technology being used. Microsoft offers information on disability access to the Internet through a special section of its website at: www.microsoft.com/enable.

Surfing the Net

Websites
There are hundreds of disability-related websites, and the number is constantly growing. The following organizations and their URLs will help you get started on the web. Happy surfing!

318

———

Computer
Resources
for People
with
Disabilities

Alliance for Technology Access

www.ATAccess.org

Includes a broad range of resource information, including The HUB, an interactive information service on disability-related products, companies, and service providers.

AbleData

www.abledata.com

A database of the full range of assistive-technology products.

Ability Hub

www.abilityhub.com

Provides information on adaptive equipment and alternative methods for accessing computers.

Disability Resources on the Internet

www.ups.edu/otpt/Disability_Info/home.html

EASI (Equal Access to Software and Information)

www.rit.edu/~easi

Family Center on Technology and Disability

www.fctd.info

Serves organizations and programs that work with families of children and youth with disabilities. Offers a range of information and services on the subject of assistive technology. The Family Center on Technology and Disability is a project of the Academy for Educational Development.

Rehabilitation Engineering and Assistive Technology Society of North America (RESNA)

www.resna.org

Tech Connections

www.techconnections.org

A collaborative project of the United Cerebral Palsy Associations, the Center for Assistive Technology and Environmental Access at the Georgia Institute of Technology, and the Southeast Disability and Business Technical Assistance Center.

The International Center for Disability Resources on the Internet (ICDRI)

www.icdri.org/WebAccess/webable.htm

Trace Research and Development Center

www.trace.wisc.edu

University of Washington
www.washington.edu/doit

Yahoo's Disability Resources
http://dir.yahoo.com/society_and_culture/disabilities

Inventories (lists of traits, skills, preferences, etc., compiled by an individual's responses to certain questions) that can be completed online provide one way to identify your learning strengths. A few examples include:

Abiator's Online Learning Styles Inventory
www.berghuis.co.nz/abiator/lsi/lsiframe.html

Center for the Advancement of Learning: Learning Strategies Database
http://muskingum.edu/~cal/database/psinventory.html

The Learning Disabilities Resource Community
www.ldrc.ca/projects/miinventory/mitest.html

Multiple Intelligences Kids Page
www.atc.unh.edu/~fisk/MIKids.html

Visit your favorite websites frequently; they are updated often and will provide valuable and current information.

In addition to World Wide Web sites, many other formats on the Internet offer innumerable resources on virtually any topic of interest to you. Different formats include news groups, bulletin boards, listserves, and discussion lists. As is the case with the World Wide Web, the number of new resources in these other formats is growing rapidly, creating unbelievable amounts of information and fostering connections with helpful, knowledgeable people.

Listserves and Discussion Lists

Listserves generally provide e-mail messages for their subscribers from other subscribers. Many listserves enable people to read archives and to receive postings over a period of time in a form called a *digest*. Before signing up for a listserve, you may want to visit its archives and review the requirements and contents of the site.

Listed below are a few listserves and discussion lists of interest to people with disabilities.

Act is an EASI Digest list for adaptive computer professionals. To subscribe, send a message with a blank subject line to listserv@maelstrom.stjohns.edu. In the body of the message type, "subscribe act [your first name] [your last name]," inserting your name where it is requested

320

Computer
Resources
for People
with
Disabilities

ADA Disability Access Issues Discussion List

ADA-ACCESS@listserv.AOL.com

AToutcomes supports the development and use of reliable, valid, and sensitive outcome measures in assistive technology. To subscribe, send a message with a blank subject line to majordomo@snow.utoronto.ca. In the body of the message type "subscribe atoutcomes [your e-mail-address]," inserting your e-mail address where it is requested. Or visit their website.

www.utoronto.ca/atrc/reference/atoutcomes/ATOListserv.html.

Axslib-l focuses on issues surrounding access to libraries by people with disabilities. It sponsors **Libraries Without Walls Discussion List (Axslib-l)**. To subscribe, send a message with a blank subject line to listserv@maelstrom.stjohns.edu. In the body of the message, type, "subscribe axslib [your first name] [your last name]," inserting your name where it is requested. Visit its website at:

www.rit.edu/~easi/lib/axslib-l.html

Blind-DEV is dedicated to the discussion of issues concerning the development of computer products and adaptive equipment for blind and visually impaired computer users. To subscribe, send a message with a blank subject line to listserv@maelstrom.stjohns.edu. In the body of the message, type, "subscribe blind-dev [your first name] [your last name]," inserting your name where it is requested. Visit its website at:

www.cs.tcd.ie/blind-dev

The **BlindFam** mailing list is for discussions of all aspects of family life as they are affected by the blindness of one or more family members. All family members are invited to join, and people are encouraged to send descriptions of themselves and their families. To subscribe to BlindFam, send an e-mail message to listserv@sjuvm.stjohns.edu or visit BlindFam's website.

http://maelstrom.stjohns.edu/archives/blindfam.html

CataList is a catalog of listserve lists. From its website, you can browse any of the 73,058 public listserve lists on the Internet, search for mailing lists of interest, and get information about listserve host sites.

www.lsoft.com/lists/listref.html

Crt-focus is for discussion of assistive technology for people with disabilities. To subscribe, send a message with a blank subject line to listproc@smash.gatech.edu. In the body of the message, type, "subscribe crt-focus [your first name] [your last name]," inserting your name where it is requested.

Deaf.Com offers several discussion groups, chat rooms, and a monthly newsletter. Access these resources by visiting its website.

www.deaf.com

The **Deaf Discussion List** provides *Deaf Magazine* to subscribers. Send an e-mail message to deaf-request@clark.net. Leave the subject line blank, and in the body of the message type, "SUB DEAF [your first name] [your last name]," inserting your name where it is requested.

DeafNotes.Com is Deaf.com's message-board site. It's a free public forum where participants can discuss controversial issues and topics of interest to the deaf community. There are several forums focusing on issues from a deaf perspective, as well as departments for "just-for-fun" postings. All forums are moderated.

Design-for-all provides an electronic platform for people who are interested in design that is accessible for everyone. For more information visit its website at:

www.design-for-all.org

EASI (Equal Access to Software and Information) deals with issues related to technology and people with disabilities. To join, send a message with a blank subject line to listserv@stuvm.stjohns.edu. In the body of the message, type, "subscribe easi [your first name] [your last name]," inserting your name where it is requested. To post to the list, send a message to

easi@sjuvm.stjohns.edu.

Freedom Scientific Users lists. Freedom Scientific, manufacturer of a wide range of assistive-technology products, helps users of its products connect to one another through its website.

www.freedomscientific.com/fs_support/User_Groups.asp

Ibm-srd is for sharing information about using IBM ScreenReader software. To subscribe, send a message with a blank subject line to listserv@vm1.-nodak.edu. In the body of the message, type, "subscribe ibm-srd [your first name] [your last name]," inserting your name where it is requested.

Information, Technology and Disabilities is a quarterly electronic journal devoted to computer use by people with disabilities. To join the list, which sends out complete issues, send a message with a blank subject line to listserv@maelstrom.stjohns.edu. In the body of the message type "SUB itd-jnl [your first name] [your last name]," inserting your name where it is requested.

322

Computer
Resources
for People
with
Disabilities

LD-List (Learning-Disability Discussion List) is an open, unmoderated, international forum that provides information for individuals interested in learning disabilities. Subscribers include people with learning disabilities, family members and friends, educators and administrators, researchers, and others wishing to know more about the subject. For more information visit its website.

www.ldresources.com

The **QIAT** (The Quality Indicators for Assistive Technology) listserv provides opportunities for participation in the process of identifying, disseminating, and implementing a set of widely applicable Quality Indicators for Assistive Technology Services in School settings. It is also a tool for consumers, family members, educators, and other professionals to share information, strategies, and experiences in their roles in the delivery and use of assistive technology services.

http://sweb.uky.edu/~jszaba0/QIAT.html

Voice-users is a discussion list for people using, or planning to use, voice recognition software. Visit its website at:

www.voicerecognition.com/voice-users

Technology Vendors

The following list indicates vendors and developers in the field today. This list is not exhaustive but represents many of the products currently available. Contact vendors directly for a full list of their products. Many of the vendors included on this list are members of the Alliance for Technology Access (indicated by an asterisk). The Alliance for Technology Access is a growing organization with new vendor members joining regularly. If you are interested in becoming a vendor member of the Alliance for Technology Access, please contact it for information and an application.

3M Touch Systems
7025 W. Marcia Rd.   (866) 407-6666
Milwaukee WI 53223   (414) 365-3555
E-mail: touch@mmm.com   (414) 365-1133, fax
Website: www.3m.com/3mtouchsystems
- Touch screens
- Monitor additions/add-ons

ABBYY USA
3823 Spinnaker Ct.   (510) 226-6717

Fremont CA 94538
E-mail: abbyyusa.com
Website: sales@abbyyusa.com

(510) 226-6069, fax

- OCR software

Ability Research, Inc.
PO Box 1721
Minnetonka MN 55345
E-mail: ability@skypoint.com
Website: www.skypoint.com/~ability

(952) 939-0121
(952) 890-8393, fax

- Augmentative and alternative communication products
- Switches

AbleLink Technologies
528 North Tejon St., Suite 100
Colorado Springs CO 80903
E-mail: support@assess.net
Website: www.ablelinktech.com

(719) 592-0347
(719) 592-0348, fax

- Accessible browsers and add-ons

*AbleNet, Inc.
1081 Tenth Ave. SE
Minneapolis MN 55414
E-mail: customerservice@ablenetinc.com
Website: www.ablenetinc.com

(800) 322-0956
(612) 379-0956, outside U.S./Canada
(612) 379-9143, fax

- Augmentative and alternative communication products
- Electronic aids to daily living
- Interface devices
- Literacy products
- Curriculum guides
- Switches
- Interface devices

*Academic Software, Inc.
3504 Tates Creek Rd.
Lexington KY 40517
E-mail: asistaff@acsw.com
Website: www.acsw.com

(859) 552-1020
(859) 273-1943, fax

- Interface devices
- Switch software
- Adaptive-device locator system

*Access First!
(See TASH International, Inc.)

324

Computer
Resources
for People
with
Disabilities

Access Solutions
4536 Edison Ave.
Sacramento CA 95821
E-mail: info@axsol.com
Website: www.axsol.com

(916) 481-3559
(916) 482-2250, fax

- Speech synthesizers

Active Words Systems, Inc.
PO Box 1251
Winter Park FL 32790
E-mail: support@activewords.com
Website: www.activewords.com

- Abbreviation expansion programs

AccuCorp, Inc.
PO Box 66
Christiansburg VA 24073

(703) 961-2001

- Chording keyboards

ADAMLAB, LLC
55 East Long Lake Rd., Suite 337
Troy MI 48085
E-mail: customerservice@adamlab.com
Website: www.adamlab.com

(248) 362-9603
(248) 362-9606, fax

- Augmentative and alternative communication products

*Adaptivation, Inc.
2225 W. 50th St., Suite 100
Sioux Falls SD 57105
E-mail: info@adaptivation.com
Website: www.adaptivation.com

(800) 723-2783
(605) 335-4445
(605) 335-4446, fax

- Augmentative and alternative communication products
- Switches and switch software

*ADAS, LLC
2728 South Cole Rd.
Boise ID 83709
E-mail: adas@ad-as.com
Website: www.ad-as.com

(800) 208-2020
(208) 362-8001
(208) 362-8009, fax

- Accessible furniture

*Ai Squared
PO Box 669
Manchester Center VT 05255-0669
E-mail: sales@aisquared.com

(802) 362-3612
(802) 362-1670, fax

Website: www.aisquared.com
- Screen magnification programs

ALDs, Inc.
4611 No. 6 Rd., Unit #220   (604) 244-0269
Richmond BC V6V 2L3   (604) 244-0024, fax
Canada
E-mail: sales@alds.com
Website: www.alds.com
- Assistive listening devices

AliMed, Inc.
297 High St.   (800) 225-2610
Dedham MA 02026   (781) 329-2900
E-mail: info@alimed.com   (800) 437-2966 toll-free fax
Website: www.alimed.com   (781) 329-8392, fax
- Arm and wrist supports

*AlphaSmart, Inc.
973 University Ave.   (888) 274-0680
Los Gatos CA 95032   (408) 355-1000
E-mail: info@alphasmart.com   (408) 355-1055, fax
- Note takers

*ALVA Access Group, Inc.
436 14th St., Suite 700   (888) 318-2582
Oakland CA 94612   (510) 451-0878, fax
E-mail: info@aagi.com
Website: www.aagi.com
- Screen readers
- Braille displays
- Screen enlargement programs
- Graphics-to-Braille representations software
- Handheld organizers

*AMDi
200 Frank Rd.   (888) 353-2634
Hicksville NY 11801   (516) 822-6611, fax
E-mail: info@amdi.net
Website: www.amdi.net
- Augmentative and alternative communication products
- Head-pointing devices
- Software
- Switches
- Mounting systems

326

Computer
Resources
for People
with
Disabilities

America Online
PO Box 10810
Herndon VA 20170
E-mail: support@aol.net
Website: www.corp.aol.com
- Internet service provider

(800) 827-6364

American Printing House for the Blind, Inc.
1839 Frankfort Ave.
PO Box 6085
Louisville KY 40206
E-mail: info@aph.org
Website: www.aph.org
- Note takers
- Screen readers
- Speech synthesizers
- Talking software

(800) 223-1839
(502) 895-2405
(502) 899-2274, fax

*American Thermoform Corporation
1758 Brackett St.
La Verne CA 91750
E-mail: atc@atcbrleqp.com
Website: www.atcbrleqp.com
- Braille embossers, translators
- Refreshable Braille displays
- Tactile graphics production

(800) 331-3676
(909) 593-6711
(909) 593-8001, fax

Ameriphone, Inc.
12082 Western Ave.
Garden Grove CA 92841-2913
E-mail: ameriphonecs@plantronics.com
Website: www.ameriphone.com
- TTY

(800) 874-3005
(800) 772-2889, TTY
(800) 897-4703, fax

*Antarq
Fernando No. 90, Col. Alamos
C.P. 03400
Mexico, D.F.
E-mail: antarq@terra.com.mx
Website: www.antarq.com.mx (bilingual Spanish/English)
- Screen readers
- Access utilities
- Screen magnification software
- Augmentative and alternative communication products

+55-19-64-97
+55-30-00-43, fax

- Abbreviation expansion and macro programs
- Access utilities
- Alternate keyboards
- Switch software
- Talking and large-print word processors
- Touch screens
- Word Prediction Programs

*Apple Computer, Inc.

Worldwide Disability Solutions   (800) 767-2775
1 Infinite Loop
Cupertino CA 95014
Website: www.apple.com/disability

- Access utilities
- Menu-management programs
- Screen magnification programs
- Voice recognition

Applied Future Technologies, Inc.

11615 W. 75th Ave.   (303) 403-0457
Arvada CO 80005   (303) 420-8817, fax
E-mail: aft@appliedfuture.com
Website: www.appliedfuture.com

- Electronic aids to daily living

*Applied Human Factors, Inc.

PO Box 228   (210) 408-0098
Helotes TX 78023   (210) 408-0097, fax
E-mail: sales@ahf-net.com
Website: www.ahf-net.com

- On-screen keyboards
- Word prediction programs

Artic Technologies-Simply Computers

1000 John R. Rd., Suite 108   (248) 588-7370
Troy MI 48083   (248) 588-2650, fax
E-mail: info@artictech.com
Website: www.artictech.com

- Screen magnification programs
- Screen readers
- Speech synthesizers

*AssisTech, Inc.

PO Box 137   (716) 789-4197
Stow NY 14785   (716) 789-4644, fax

TECHNOLOGY VENDORS / A

328

Computer
Resources
for People
with
Disabilities

E-mail: info@assisttech.com
Website: www.assisttech.com
- Early-childhood products
- Educational technology
- Computer keyboards
- Keyguards

*Assistive Technology, Inc.

7 Wells Ave.	(800) 793-9227
Newton MA 02459	(617) 641-9000
E-mail: customercare@assistivetech.com	(617) 641-9191, fax

Website: www.assistivetech.com
- Alternative and augmentative communication products
- Authoring software
- Speech synthesizers
- Alternate input
- Processing aids
- Switch software

AT&T Wireless

Website: www.attwireless.com	(800) 888-7600

- Cell phones
- TTY
- TTY modems and software
- Video relay service

*Attainment Company

PO Box 930160	(800) 327-4269
504 Commerce Pkwy.	(800) 942-3865, fax
Verona WI 53593	

E-mail: info@attainmentcompany.com
Website: www.attainmentcompany.com
- Augmentative and alternative communication products
- Electronic **aids** to daily living
- Parent resources
- Professional resources
- Academic software

*Aurora Systems, Inc.

Box 43005	(888) 290-1133
Burnaby BC V5G 3H0	(604) 291-6310
Canada	(604) 291-6310, fax

E-mail: service@aurora-systems.com
Website: www.aurora-systems.com

- Alternative and augmentative communication products
- Processing aids
- Word prediction programs

BAUM Retec AG

Schloss Langenzell   +49-6223-4909-0
69257 Wiesenbach   +49-6223-4909-99, fax
Germany
E-mail: info@baum.de
Website: www.baum.de
- Reading machines
- Access utilities

Bellaire Electronics

4 Broadgate   +44-0-1271-324759
Bellaire, Barnstaple   +44-0-870-164-1193, fax
Devon EX31 1QZ
UK
E-mail: chris@bellaire.co.uk
Website: www.bellaire.co.uk
- Chording keyboard

The Benetech Initiative

480 S. California Ave., Suite 201   (650) 475-5440
Palo Alto CA 94306-1609   (650) 475-1066, fax
E-mail: info@benetech.org
Website: www.benetech.org
- Online library of accessible digital books (www.Bookshare.org)
- Martus human-rights bulletin system

*Betacom Corporation

450 Matheson Blvd. E., Suite 67   (800) 353-1107, ext. 230
Mississauga ON L4Z 1R5   (905) 658-9925
Canada
E-mail: info@betacom.com
Website: www.betacom.com
- CCTVs
- Visual aids

Beyond Sight, Inc.

5650 South Windermere St.   (303) 795-6455
Littleton CO 80120   (303) 795-6425, fax
Website: www.beyondsight.com
- Braille embossers and translators
- CCTVs

330

Computer
Resources
for People
with
Disabilities

- Screen magnification programs
- Screen readers
- Speech synthesizers

Biolink Computer Research and Development, Ltd.
4770 Glenwood Ave.   (604) 984-4099
North Vancouver BC V7R 4G8   (604) 985-7114, fax
Canada
E-mail: sales@biolink.bc.ca
Website: www.biolink.bc.ca
- Screen readers

Blissymbolics Communication International
1630 Lawrence Ave. W., Suite 104   (416) 242-9114
Toronto ON M6L 3C5   (416) 244-6543, fax
Canada
E-mail: klseybold@sympatico.ca
Website: http://home.istar.ca/~bci
- Writing-composition programs

*Boost Technology
1601 Ocean Ave.   (866) BOOST HELP (266-7843)
San Francisco CA 94112-1717
E-mail: ata@boosttechnology.com
Website: www.boosttechnology.com
- Electronic head-pointing device

Brain Actuated Technologies, Inc.
1350 President St.   (937) 767-2674
Yellow Springs OH 45387   (937) 767-7366, fax
E-mail: support@brainfingers.com
Website: www.brainfingers.com
- Electronic pointing devices

Brainium Technologies Inc.
Corporate Headquarters   (800) 663-7163
11491 Kingston St.   (877) 373-2697, fax
Maple Ridge BC V2X 0Y6
Canada
E-mail: info@brainium.com
Website: www.brainium.com
- Note takers

BrainTrain, Inc.
727 Twin Ridge Ln.   (800) 822-0538

Richmond VA 23235   (804) 320-0105
E-mail: info@braintrain.com   (804) 320-0242, fax
Website: www.braintrain.com
- Cognitive-training software

*Brøderbund Software, Inc.
(see Riverdeep, Inc.)

Bytes of Learning
60 Renfrew Dr., Suite 210   (800) 465-6428
Markham ON L3R OE1   (905) 947-4646
Canada   (905) 475-8650, fax
E-mail: custservice@bytesoflearning.com
Website: www.bytesoflearning.com
- Talking word processors
- Educational software

Cables to Go
1501 Webster St.   (937) 224-8646
Dayton OH 45404   (800) 331-2841, fax
E-mail: customer-service@cablestogo.com
Website: www.cablestogo.com
- Monitor additions

CAD & Graphics
1161 Chess Dr., Suite D   (888) 686-0551
Foster City CA 94404   (650) 627-0015
Website: www.cadandgraphics.com
- OCR software

Carolyn's Products for Enhanced Living
PO Box 14577   (800) 648-2266
Bradenton FL 34208   (941) 739-5503, fax
E-mail: sales@carolynscatalog.com
Website: www.carolynscatalog.com
- CCTVs
- Keyboard add-ons
- Monitor additions

Cellular One
Website: www.cellularone.com   (800) 828-0507
- Cell phones

*Center for Applied Special Technology (CAST)
40 Harvard Mills Sq., Suite 3   (781) 245-2212
Wakefield MA 01880-3233

332

Computer
Resources
for People
with
Disabilities

E-mail: cast@cast.org
Website: www.cast.org
- Educational software
- Reading comprehension programs
- Talking and large-print word processors

CE Software, Inc.
PO Box 65580   (800) 523-7638
West Des Moines IA 50265   (515) 221-1801
E-mail: sales@cesoft.com   (515) 221-1806, fax
Website: www.cesoft.com
- Abbreviation expansion and macro programs

Cingular
Website: www.cingular.com   (800) 331-0500
- Cell phones

Cirque Corporation
2463 South 3850 West, Suite A   (800) 454-3375
Salt Lake City UT 84120   (801) 467-1100
Website: www.cirque.com   (801) 467-0208, fax
- Trackballs

*Clarity Solutions
6409 Alisal St.   (800) 575-1456
Pleasanton CA 94566   (925) 484-3801, fax
E-mail: clarity@clarityusa.com
Website: www.clarityusa.com
- CCTVs

*Closing the Gap, Inc.
PO Box 68   (507) 248-3294
526 Main St.   (507) 248-3810, fax
Henderson MN 56044
E-mail: info@closingthegap.com
Website: www.closingthegap.com
- Information resources

Code-It Software, Inc.
PO Box 171   (307) 437-6629
Midwest WY 82643   (307) 437-6629, fax
E-mail: mikeB@code-it.com
Website: www.code-it.com
- Accessible browsers

*Cogent Systems, Inc.
10151 University Blvd., Suite 366
Orlando FL 32817
E-mail: info@cosys.com
Website: www.cosys.com
 • Cognitive software and products

*Commodio
10250 Valley View Rd., Suite 143
Eden Prairie MN 55344
E-mail: info@commodio.com
Website: www.commodio.com
 • Voice recognition

(407) 679-6377
(407) 679-0675

(800) 886-3996
(952) 944-5646, fax

Communication Skill Builders
(see Psychological Corporation)

Compass Learning
9920 Pacific Heights Blvd., Suite 500
San Diego CA 92121-4330
Website: www.compasslearning.com
 • Reading comprehension programs
 • Software features: built-in utilities
 • Talking and large-print word processors
 • Educational software

(800) 247-1380
(619) 587-0087
(619) 622-7873, fax

Compusult Limited
PO Box 1000
Mt. Pearl NF A1N 3C9
Canada
E-mail: hear-it@compusult.nf.ca
Website: www.hear-it.com
 • Speech synthesizers
 • Text-to-speech software
 • Joysticks
 • Closed-caption display units

(888) 307-7707
(709) 745-7914
(709) 745-7927, fax

*Compu-Teach
PMB 137
16541 Redmond Way, Suite C
Redmond WA 98052
E-mail: info@compu-teach.com
Website: www.compu-teach.com
 • Educational software
 • Reading comprehension programs

(800) 448-3224
(425) 885-0517
(425) 883-9169, fax

334

Computer
Resources
for People
with
Disabilities

Computers to Help People, Inc.
825 E. Johnson St.   (608) 257-5917
Madison WI 53713
Website: www.chpi.org
  • Switch software

Conover Company
2926 Hidden Hollow Rd.   (920) 231-4667
Oshkosh WI 54901   (920) 231-4809, fax
E-mail: conover@execpc.com
Website: http:www.conovercompany.com
  • Software: work-skills training

*Consultants for Communication Technology
508 Bellevue Terrace   (412) 761-6062
Pittsburgh PA 15202   (412) 761-7336, fax
E-mail: CCT@ConCommTech.com
Website: www.ConCommTech.com
  • Elextronic aids to daily living
  • Switch-interface devices
  • Speech synthesizers
  • Switch software

Continental Press, Inc.
520 East Bainbridge St.   (800) 233-0759
Elizabethtown PA 17022
E-mail: cpeducation@continentalpress.com
Website: www.continentalpress.com
  • Reading comprehension programs

Corel, Inc.
8144 Walnut Hill Ln., Suite 1050   (800) 772-6735
Dallas TX 75231   (613) 761-9176, fax
E-mail: custserv@corel.com
Website: www.corel.com
  • Abbreviation expansion and macros
  • Large-print word processors

CPR Technology
640 Dean St.   (718) 783-6000
Brooklyn NY 11238
E-mail: cpr@cprtech.com
Website: www.cprtech.com
  • Pagers

*Creative Communicating
PO Box 3358
Park City UT 84060
E-mail: mail@creative-comm.com
Website: www.creative-comm.com

(435) 645-7737
(435) 658-0925, fax

- Early-learning products
- Literacy materials
- Educational software

Creative Learning Company
PO Box 106239
Downtown Auckland
New Zealand
E-mail: info@clc.co.nz
Website: www.creativelearningcentre.com

+64-9-309-3701
+64-9-309-3708, fax

- Reading comprehension programs

Crestwood Communication Aids, Inc.
6625 N. Sydney Pl., Dept. 21F
Milwaukee WI 53209-3259
E-mail: crestcomm@aol.com
Website: www.communicationaids.com

(414) 352-5678
(414) 352-5679, fax

- Augmentative and alternative communication products
- Pointing and typing aids

*Crick Software
50 116th Ave. SE, Suite 211
Bellevue WA 98004
E-mail: info@cricksoft.com
Website: www.cricksoft.com

(866) 33-CRICK (332-7425)
(425) 467-8260
(425) 467-8245

- Reading comprehension programs
- Writing-composition programs
- On-screen keyboards
- Switch-interface devices

Data Cal Corporation, LLC
1345 N. Mondel Dr.
Gilbert AZ 85233
Website: www.datacal.com

(800) 223-0123
(480) 813-3100
(480) 545-8090, fax

- Keyboard add-ons

DeafNation
PO Box 762
Frederick MD 21705
E-mail: info@deafnation.com

(301) 682-7529, fax

Website: www.deafnation.com
- Pagers

336

Computer
Resources
for People
with
Disabilities

DeafWorks
PO Box 1265   (800) 855-2881, voice relay (USA)
Provo UT 84603-1265   (888) 735-5906, in state
E-mail: info@deafworks.com   (801) 465-1957, TTY
Website: www.deafworks.com   (801) 465-1958, fax
- TTY

*Digital Frog International
Trillium Pl.   (519) 766-1097
7377 Calfass Rd. RR #2   (519) 767-9994
Puslinch ON N0B 2J0
Canada
E-mail: info@digitalfrog.com
Website: www.digitalfrog.com
- Accessible science software

Discis Knowledge Research, Inc.
90 Sheppard Ave. E., 7th Fl.   (416) 250-6537
Toronto ON M2N 3A1   (416) 250-6540, fax
Canada
E-mail: discis@goodmedia.com
Website: www.goodmedia.com/discis
- Reading comprehension programs

*Dolphin Computer Access
60 East Third Ave., Suite 130   (866) 797-5921
San Mateo CA 94401   (650) 348 7403, fax
E-mail: info@dolphinusa.com
Website: www.dolphinuk.co.uk
- Braille output
- Screen reader
- Screen magnification programs

*Don Johnston, Inc.
26799 W. Commerce Dr.   (800) 999-4660
Volo IL 60073   (847) 740-0749
E-mail: info@donjohnston.com   (847) 740-7326, fax
Website: www.donjohnston.com
- Augmentative and alternative communication products
- Reading comprehension programs
- Switch software
- Talking and large-print word processors

- Word prediction programs
- Writing-composition programs
- Literacy programs
- Switches
- Mounting systems
- Curriculum guides
- Interface devices

DS Ergonomics
Gates House 111-113 Fortis GN +44-0-20-8883-6421
London N29 HR +44-0-20-8883-6194, fax
UK
E-mail: info@datasound.com
Website: www.datasound.com
- Arm and wrist supports

*DU-IT Control Systems Group, Inc.
(see GenesisOne Technologies Inc.)
- Electronic aids to daily living
- Switches and switch software

*Dunamis, Inc.
3545 Cruse Rd., Suite 312 (770) 279-1144
Lawrenceville GA 30044 (770) 279-0809, fax
E-mail: info@dunamisinc.com
Website: www.dunamisinc.com
- Communication-skills software
- Educational software
- Alternate input

DuPont Displays
14 T.W. Alexander Dr. (919) 248-5031
PO Box 13999 (919) 248-5219, fax
Research Triangle Park NC 27709
Website: www.dupont.com/displays
- Antiglare screens

Duxbury Systems, Inc.
270 Littleton Rd., Unit 6 (978) 692-3000
Westford MA 01886-3523 (978) 692-7912, fax
E-mail: info@duxsys.com
Website: www.duxburysystems.com
- Braille editing software
- Braille embossers, translators
- Screen readers
- Speech synthesizers

338

Computer
Resources
for People
with
Disabilities

*DynaVox Systems
2100 Wharton St., Suite 400   (800) 344-1778
Pittsburgh PA 15203   (412) 381-4883
E-mail: contact@dynavoxsys.com   (412) 381-5241, fax
Website: www.dynavoxsys.com
  • Augmentative and alternative communication products
  • Electronic aids to daily living

Eco-Net International
110404 Lakeview Dr.   (954) 345-0213
Coral Springs FL 33071
E-mail: Ammirata@econointl.com
Website: www.econointl.com
  • Accessible browsers and add-ons

EDCON Publishing Group
30 Montauk Blvd.   (888) 553-3266
Oakdale NY 11769   (631) 567-7227
E-mail: info@edconpublishing.com   (631) 567-8745, fax
Website: www.edconpublishing.com
  • Educational software

Edmark
(see Riverdeep, Inc.)

Educational Activities, Inc.
PO Box 87   (800) 645-3739
Baldwin NY 11510   (516) 623-9282, fax
E-mail: learn@edact.com
Website: www.edact.com
  • Reading comprehension programs
  • Educational software

*Education TURNKEY Systems, Inc.
256 North Washington St.   (703) 536-2310
Falls Church VA 22046   (703) 536-3225, fax
E-mail: turnkey@ix.netcom.com
Website: www.edturnkey.com
  • Consulting services

EKEG Electronics Company, Ltd.
26227 62nd Ave.   (866) 721-EKEG (721-3534)
Aldergrove BC V4W 1L8   (604) 857-0828
Canada   (604) 857-2726, fax
E-mail: ekeg@ekegelectronics.com

Website: www.ekegelectronics.com
- Alternate keyboards

Elan Speech

3939 La Lauragaise   +33-5-62-24-71-00
BP 758   +33-5-62-24-71-01, fax
31683 Labege Cedex
France
E-mail: info@elanspeech.com
Website: www.elantts.com
- Speech synthesizer

Enabling Devices and Toys for Special Children

385 Warburton Ave.   (800) TEC-TOYS (832-8697)
Hastings-on-Hudson NY 10706   (914) 478-0960
E-mail: info@enablingdevices.com   (914) 478-7030, fax
Website: www.enablingdevices.com
- Communication aids
- Keyboard additions
- Switches and switch software
- Adapted toys
- Electronic aids to daily living

Enabling Technologies Company

1601 Northeast Braille Pl.   (800) 777-3687 (U.S. only)
Jensen Beach FL 34957   (772) 225-3687
Website: www.brailler.com   (772) 225-3299, fax (U.S. only)
- Braille embossers and translators

Enhanced Vision, Inc.

17911 Sampson Ln.   (888) 811-3161
Huntington Beach CA 92647   (714) 374-1829
E-mail: info@enhancedvision.com   (714) 374-1821, fax
Website: www.enhancedvision.com
- CCTVs

*Enkidu Research, Inc.

17800 W. Capitol Dr.   (800) 297-9570
Brookfield WI 53045   (716) 433-6164
E-mail: info@enkidu.net
Website: www.enkidu.net
- Augmentative and alternative communication products
- PDAs

340

Computer
Resources
for People
with
Disabilities

Epson
E-mail: support@epson.com   (800) 922-8911
Website: www.epson.com
  • Scanners

Ergo Kare
1644 Conestoga St., Suite 2   (800) 927-5273
Boulder CO 80301   (303) 443-4243
E-mail: info@kareproducts.com   (303) 443-2522, fax
Website: www.kareproducts.com
  • Trackballs
  • Arm and wrist supports

*ErgoMETRIX
411 S. Main, Suite 405   (888) 700-0310
Los Angeles CA 90013   (888) 841-3711
E-mail: info@ergometrix.com
Website: www.adaptivetables.com
  • Ergonomic tables

Esselte Americas
48 South Service Rd.   (800) 645-6051
Melville NY 11747   (631) 675-5700
Website: www.esselteamericas.com   (800) 331-0231, fax
  • Computer accessories
  • Monitor mounts

*Exceller Software Corporation
10999 Reed Hartman Hwy., Suite 330   (513) 792-9555
Cincinnati OH 45242   (513) 792-9546, fax
E-mail: info@exceller.com
Website: www.exceller.com
  • Linguistic and reference software
  • Bilingual software in Spanish, Portuguese, German, and Italian

Exceptional Computing, Inc.
450 NW 58th St.   (352) 331-8847
Gainesville FL 32607   (352) 331-4164, fax
E-mail: rhm@exceptionalcomputing.com
Website: www.exceptionalcomputing.com
  • Alternate keyboards
  • Switches and switch software
  • Educational software

Extensions for Independence
555 Saturn Blvd. #B-368 (619) 423-1748
San Diego CA 92154 (866) 632-7149, voice mail, fax (U.S. only)
Website: www.mouthstick.net
- Alternate keyboards
- Pointing and typing aids

Eye Control Technologies, Inc. (dba NaturalPoint)
PO Box 2317 (541) 753-6645
Corvallis OR 97339 (541) 753-6689, fax
E-mail: sales@naturalpoint.com
Website: www.eyecontrol.com
- Electronic head-pointing devices

EyeTech Digital Systems, Inc.
1705 East McLelland Rd. (480) 610-1899
Mesa AZ 85203 (703) 814-8626, fax
E-mail: info@eyetechds.com
Website: www.eyetechds.com
- Alternative pointing

Fellowes
1789 Norwood Ave. (800) 955-0959
Itasca IL 60143
Website: www.fellowes.com
- Joysticks
- Trackballs

Fentek Industries, Inc.
470 S. Main St., Suite G (800) 639-0710
PO Box 2278 (928) 639-0161
Cottonwood AZ 86326 (928) 639-0551, fax
E-mail: inforequest@fentek-ind.com
Website: www.fentek-ind.com
- Alternate keyboards

*FileMaker, Inc.
PO Box 58168 (408) 987-7000
Santa Clara CA 95052
Website: www.filemaker.com
- Home and business software

Fliptrack OneOnOne Computer Training
2055 Army Trail Rd., Suite 100 (800) 222-3547
Addison IL 60101
- Audio training tapes

342

Computer
Resources
for People
with
Disabilities

Florida New Concepts Marketing, Inc.
PO Box 261   (727) 842-3231, phone, fax
Port Richey FL 34673-0261
E-mail: compulnz@gte.net
Website: www.gulfside.com/compulenz
  • Monitor additions/add-ons

Focused Technology
7356 South Tamiami Trail   (888) 686-0551
Sarasota FL 34231   (941) 926-0624
PO Box 17315   (941) 927-6431, fax
Sarasota FL 34276
E-mail: sales@focusedtechnology.com
Website: www.focusedtechnology.com
  • Monitor additions/add-ons

Franklin Electronic Publishers, Inc.
One Franklin Plaza   (800) 266-5626
Burlington NJ 08016   (609) 239-5948, fax
E-mail: service@franklin.com
Website: www.franklin.com
  • Electronic reference tools

*Freedom Scientific Blind/Low-Vision Group
11800 31st Court N.   (800) 444-4443
St. Petersburg FL 33716-1805   (727) 803-8000
E-mail: info@freedomscientific.com   (727) 803-8001, fax
Website: www.freedomscientific.com
  • Braille embossers
  • Braille translation software
  • Note takers
  • Screen readers
  • Screen magnification programs
  • Browser access
  • PDAs

*Freedom Scientific Learning Systems Group
480 California Ave., Suite 201   (888) 223-3344
Palo Alto CA 94036-1609   (650) 475-5435
E-mail: wynn@freedomscientific.com   (650) 475-1067, fax
Website: www.freedomscientific.com/wynn
  • Reading comprehension programs
  • Electronic reference tools
  • OCR software

*FutureForms

903 Chicago Ave.
Grand Rapids MI 49509
E-mail: info@futureforms.com
Website: www.futureforms.com

(888) 786-6455, ext. 236 or 227
(616) 475-0491, fax

- Electronic forms
- Electronic reference tools

GEWA (UK) Ltd.

8 Farmbrough Close
Stocklake
Aylesbury
Bucks HP20 1DQ
UK
E-mail: info@gewa.co.uk
Website: www.possum.co.uk/Gewa/Index.htm

+44-0-1296-461-003
+44-0-1296-461-107, fax

- Communication devices
- Electronic aids to daily living

Garmin International, Inc.

1200 E. 151st St.
Olathe KS 66062
Website: www.garmin.com

(800) 800-1020
(913) 397-8200
(913) 397-8282, fax

- Global positioning systems (GPS)

GenesisOne Technologies Inc.

794 Parkview Dr.
Wooster OH 44691
Website: www.apt-technology.com

(888) 221-5032
(330) 263-0015
(775) 252-4834, fax

- Switches
- Electronic aids to daily living

Grant Enterprises Online/Safco-ErgoComfort Computer Accessories

2510 Wigwam Pkwy., Suite 101
Henderson NV 89074
Website: www.grant-ent.com/safco/2gsc01.htm

(800) 338-5370
(877) 202-0019, fax

- Monitor additions/add-ons

Gravis

2000 Alameda de las Pulgas, 2nd Fl.
San Mateo CA 94403-1289
E-mail: custserv@gravis.com
Website: www.gravis.com

(650) 572-2700

- Joysticks

344

Computer
Resources
for People
with
Disabilities

*The Great Talking Box Company
22458 Fortune Dr., Suite A   (877) 275-4482
San Jose CA 95131   (408) 456-0133
E-mail: inquire@greattalkingbox.com   (408) 456-0134, fax
Website: www.greattalkingbox.com
   • Augmentative and alternative communication products

Great Wave Software
(see McGraw-Hill Children's Publishing)

*Gus Communications
1006 Lonetree Ct.   (866) 487-1006 (U.S. only)
Bellingham WA 98229   (360) 715-8580
E-mail: admin@gusinc.com   (360) 715-9633, fax
Website: www.gusinc.com
   • Abbreviation expansion and macro programs
   • Access utilities
   • Alternate keyboards
   • Augmentative and alternative communication products
   • Electronic aids to daily living
   • Speech synthesizers
   • Switch software
   • Switch interfaces
   • Talking and large-print word processors
   • Touch screens
   • Word prediction programs

GW Micro
725 Airport North Office Park   (219) 489-3671
Fort Wayne IN 46825   (219) 489-2608, fax
E-mail: support@gwmicro.com
Website: www.gwmicro.com
   • Braille embossers and translators
   • Screen magnification programs
   • Screen readers
   • Speech synthesizers
   • Browser access

Handykey Corporation
1565 Adams   (303) 331-0800
Denver CO 80206   (303) 331-6767, fax
E-mail: info@handykey.com
Website: www.handykey.com
   • Alternate keyboards

HARC Mercantile Ltd.

1111 West Centre Ave.
Portage MI 49024
Website: www.harcmercantile.com
- TTY
- Assistive listening devices

(800) 445-9968, voice, TTY
(269) 324-0301, voice, TTY
(800) 413-5248, fax
(269) 324-2387, fax

Harris Communications, Inc.

15155 Technology Dr.
Eden Prairie MN 55344-2277
E-mail: mail@harriscomm.com
Website: www.harriscomm.com
- TTYs
- Amplifiers
- Accessible pagers
- TTY modems
- Assistive listening devices

(800) 825-6758
(800) 825-9187, TTY
(612) 906-1099, fax

*Hartley Courseware, Inc.

(see Compass Learning)

Hatch Inc.

PO Box 11927
Winston-Salem NC 27116
E-mail: kelgreen@computersforkids.com
Website: www.hatchstuff.com
- Alternate keyboards
- Switch interfaces
- Switches
- Touch screens

(800) 624-7968
(336) 744-7280
(800) 410-7282, fax

Hear More, Inc.

42 Executive Blvd.
Farmingdale NY 11735
- TTYs

(800) 881-4327
(800) 281-3555, TTY
(631) 752-0689, fax

Hear You Are, Inc.

4 Muscontcong Ave.
Stanhope NJ 07874
- TTYs and TTY modems

(973) 347-7662, voice, TTY, fax

Hewlett-Packard Company

3000 Hanover St.
Palo Alto CA 94394-1185
Website: welcome.hp.com
- Scanners

(800) 752-0900
(650) 857-1501
(650) 857-5518, fax

346

Computer
Resources
for People
with
Disabilities

HITEC Group International
8160 S. Madison St.
Burr Ridge IL 60527
E-mail: info@hitec.com
Website: www.hitec.com
- TTYs
- Telecommunications equipment

(800) 288-8303
(800) 536-8890, TTY
(888) 654-9219, fax

Hooleon Corporation
417 South 6th St., Bldg. A
Cottonwood AZ 86326
E-mail: sales@hooleon.com
Website: www.hooleon.com
- Keyboard additions

(800) 937-1337
(928) 634-7515
(928) 634-4620, fax

Houghton Mifflin School Division: Eduplace
222 Berkeley St.
Boston MA 02116
Website: www.eduplace.com
- Reading comprehension programs
- Educational software
- Electronic reference tools

(800) 733-2828

*Humanities Software
PO Box 950
408 Columbia St.
Hood River OR 97031
E-mail: info@humanitiessoftware.com
Website: www.humantiessoftware.com
- Writing-composition programs
- Educational software

(800) 245-6737
(541) 386-6737
(541) 386-1410, fax

*IBM Accessibility Center
11400 Burnet Rd.
Austin TX 78758
Website: www-3.ibm.com/able
- Access utilities
- Screen readers
- Talking Internet browsers
- Voice recognition
- Abbreviation expansion and macros
- Speech synthesizers

(800) 426-4832

*Inclusive TLC, Inc.
315 Wootton St., Unit A

(800) 462-0930, ext. 205

Boonton NJ 07005 (973) 331-9849

E-mail: janet@inclusivetlc.com
Website: www.inclusivetlc.com
- Switches
- Switch software
- Alternate keyboards
- Augmentative and alternative communication products

*Independent Living Aids
200 Robbins Ln. (800) 537-2118
Jericho NY 11753 (516) 937-3906, fax
Website: www.independentliving.com *or* indlivaids.com
- Living aids for people with vision impairments
- Pointing and typing aids
- PDAs

Index Braille Printer Company
Hantverksvagen 20 +46-920-20-30-80
Box 155 +46-920-20-30-85, fax
S-954 23 Gammelstad
Sweden
E-mail: info@indexbraille.com
Website: www.indexbraille.com
- Braille embossers and translators

Inference Group: Dasher Project
Gatsby Charitable Foundation +44-0-20-7410-0330
Allington House (1st Fl.) +44-0-20-7410-0332, fax
150 Victoria Street
London SW1E 5AE
UK
E-mail: contact@gatsby.org.uk
Website: www.inference.phy.cam.ac.uk/dasher/SpecialNeeds.html
- On-screen keyboards

Infogrip, Inc.
1794 E. Main St. (800) 397-0921
Ventura CA 93001 (805) 652-0770
E-mail: infogrip@infogrip.com (805) 652-0880, fax
Website: www.infogrip.com
- Alternate keyboards
- Trackballs

*Information Services, Inc.
PO Box 7056 (888) 492-4925

348

Computer
Resources
for People
with
Disabilities

Water St.
St. John's NF A1E 3Y3
Canada
E-mail: sales@is-inc.com
Website: www.is-inc.com
- Writing-composition software

Innovative Designs
913 San Ramon Valley Blvd., Suite 280
Danville CA 94526
E-mail: FinishLine@FeaturedItems.com
Website: www.finishline.featureditems.com
- Word prediction programs

*Innovation Management Group, Inc.
22311 Ventura Blvd., Suite 104
Woodland Hills CA 91364
E-mail: cs@imgpresents.com
Website: www.imgpresents.com
- Mouse alternatives
- Alternate keyboard
- Screen magnification programs

(709) 737-2539, fax

(800) 889-0987
(818) 346-3581
(877) 464-7763, fax
(818) 346-3973, fax

*Innovative Products
830 South 48th St.
Grand Forks ND 58201
Website: www.iphope.com
- Mobility products for children

(800) 950-5185

Inspiration Software
7412 SW Beaverton-Hillsdale Hwy., Suite 102
Portland OR 97225
E-mail: webmaster@inspiration.com
Website: www.inspiration.com
- Writing-composition programs

(800) 877-4292
(503) 297-3004
(503) 297-4676, fax

Institute for Disabilities Research and Training, Inc.
11323 Amherst Ave.
Silver Spring MD 20902
E-mail: idrtorder@idrt.com
Website: www.idrt.com
- TTY modems and software

(301) 942-4326, voice, TTY
(301) 942-4439, fax

Intelligent Products
91 Dartmouth St.
Marlborough MA 01752

(508) 251-1308

E-mail: sales@softtty.com
Website: www.softtty.com
- TTY modems and software

*IntelliTools
1720 Corporate Circle   (800) 899-6687
Petaluma CA 94954   (707) 773-2000
E-mail: info@intellitools.com   (707) 773-2001, fax
Website: www.intellitools.com
- Access utilities
- Alternate keyboards
- Keyboard additions
- Switch software
- Talking and large-print word processors
- Educational software
- Curriculum software
- Interface devices
- Writing-composition software

InterAct Plus
2225 Drake Ave., Suite 2   (800) 944-8002
Huntsville AL 35805   (256) 704-8787
E-mail: info@interactplus.com   (256) 880-8785, fax
- Electronic aids to daily living

*In Touch Systems
11 Westview Rd.   (800) 332-6244
Spring Valley NY 10977   (845) 354-7431
E-mail: susanc@magicwandkeyboard.com
Website: www.magicwandkeyboard.com
- Alternate keyboards

ION Systems
107 Mississippi Ave.   (800) 983-6397
Crystal City MO 63019   (636) 937-9094
Website: www.ionwebeyes.com
- Accessible browsers and add-ons

Jbliss Imaging Systems
100 W. El Camino Real, Suite 68   (888) 4JBLISS (452-5477)
Mountain View CA 94040   (650) 940-4115
E-mail: info@jbliss.com   (650) 903-4136, fax
Website: www.jbliss.com/corporate
- Reading machines
- Accessible browsers and add-ons

350

Computer
Resources
for People
with
Disabilities

*Judy Lynn Software
PO Box 373
East Brunswick NJ 08816
E-mail: techsupt@judylynn.com
Website: www.judylynn.com

(732) 390-8845, phone/fax

- Switch software

K–12 MicroMedia Publishing
16 McKee Dr.
Mahwah NJ 07430
E-mail: sales@k12mmp.com
Website: www.k12mmp.com

(800) 292-1997
(201) 529-4500
(201) 529-5282, fax

- Educational software
- Reading comprehension programs

Kare Products/Ergo Kare, Inc.
1644 Conestoga St., Suite 2
Boulder CO 80301
E-mail: info@kareproducts.com
Website: www.kareproducts.com

(800) 927-5273
(303) 443-4243
(303) 443-2522, fax

- Arm and wrist supports
- Ergonomic products

Kensington
2000 Alameda de las Pulgas, 2nd Fl.
San Mateo CA 94403-1289
Website: www.kensington.com

(800) 235-6708
(650) 572-2700
(650) 577-0595, fax

- Joysticks
- Gaming devices
- Monitor additions: antiglare filters
- Trackballs
- Mouse alternatives/emulators

*Keyboard Alternatives & Vision Solutions
365A Tesconi Circle
Santa Rosa CA 95401
E-mail: keyalt@keyalt.com
Website: www.keyalt.com

(800) 953-9262
(707) 544-8000
(707) 522-1343, fax

- Screen magnification programs
- Ergonomic products
- Programmable keyboards
- Braille output
- Arm and wrist supports

*Keybowl, Inc.
206 S. Park Ave.   (407) 622-7774
Winter Park FL 32789
E-mail: info@keybowl.com
Website: www.keybowl.com
- Alternate keyboards

Keytec, Inc.
1293 N. Plano Rd.   (800) 624-4289 (U.S.)
Richardson TX 75081   (972) 234-8617
E-mail: sales@magictouch.com   (972) 234-8542, fax
Website: www.MAGICTOUCH.com
- Touch screens

Keytools Ltd.
PO Box 700   +44-23-8058-4314
Southampton SO17 1LQ   +44-23-8055-6902, fax
UK
E-mail: info@keytools.com
Website: www.keytools.com
- Trackballs
- Keyguards

Knowledge Adventure/Vivendi Games
6080 Center Dr., 10th Fl.   (800) 545-7667
Los Angeles CA 90045   (310) 431-4000
Website: www.vugames.com/studio.do?studioName=Knowledge_Adventure
- Reading comprehension programs
- Writing-composition software

Kurzweil Educational Systems, Inc.
14 Crosby Dr.   (800) 894-5374
Bedford MA 01730-1402   (781) 276-0600
E-mail: info@kurzweiledu.com   (781) 276-0650
Website: www.kurzweiledu.com
- Reading comprehension programs
- OCR software
- Reading machines

KY Enterprises
3025 E. 2nd St.   (562) 433-5244
Long Beach CA 90803   (562) 433-3970, fax
E-mail: info@quadcontrol.com
Website: www.quadcontrol.com

352

Computer
Resources
for People
with
Disabilities

- Electronic aids to daily living
- Joysticks
- Switches

Lake Software
E-mail: CNT@lakefolks.com
Website: www.lakefolks.com
- On-screen keyboards

*Laureate Learning Systems, Inc.
110 East Spring St.   (800) 562-6801
Winooski VT 05404   (802) 655-4755
- Educational software
- Reading comprehension programs
- Switch software
- Writing-composition programs

*Lawrence Productions
1800 South 35th St.   (800) 421-4157
Galesburg MI 49053   (616) 665-7075
- Educational Software   (616) 665-7060, fax
- Electronic aids to daily living

*LC Technologies, Inc.
9455 Silver King Ct.   (800) 393-4293
Fairfax VA 22031   (703) 385-7133
E-mail: info@eyegaze.com   (703) 385-7137, fax
Website: www.eyegaze.com
- Alternate input
- Electronic aids to daily living

*LD Resources
202 Lake Rd.   (860) 868-3214
New Preston CT 06777
E-mail: richard@ldresources.com
Website: www.ldresources.com
- Consulting services
- Educational software

The Learning Company
(see Riverdeep, Inc.)

*Learning Well
111 Kane St.   (800) 645-6564
Baltimore MD 21224   (800) 413-7442, fax
E-mail: learningwell@wclm.com

Website: www.learningwelled.com
- Educational software

Less Gauss, Inc.
1164 Route 9G
Hyde Park NY 12538
E-mail: info@lessgauss.com
Website: www.lessgauss.com
- Arm and wrist supports
- Monitor additions: magnifiers

(877) 828-4817
(845) 229-1715, fax

Lexia Learning Systems, Inc.
114 Lewis St.
Lincoln MA 01773
E-mail: info@lexialearning.com
Website: www.lexialearning.com
- Reading comprehension programs

(800) 435-3942
(781) 259-8752
(781) 259-1349, fax

Little Planet Learning
(see Sunburst Technology Corporation)

Logitech, Inc.
6505 Kaiser Dr.
Fremont CA 94555
Website: www.logitech.com
- Trackballs
- Joysticks

(800) 231-7717
(510) 795-8500

*LS&S
PO Box 673
Northbrook IL 60065
E-mail: info@LSSproducts.com
Website: www.lssgroup.com
- CCTVs
- Visual aids
- TTYs
- Products for the deaf and hearing impaired

(800) 468-4789
(847) 498-9777
(866) 317-8533, TTY, TDD
(847) 498-1482, fax

Luminaud, Inc.
8688 Tyler Blvd.
Mentor OH 44060
E-mail: info@luminaud.com
Website: www.luminaud.com
- Augmentative and alternative communication products
- Switches and switch software

(800) 255-3408
(440) 255-9082
(440) 255-2250, fax

354

Computer
Resources
for People
with
Disabilities

*Lynjan Solutions, LLC
51158 Garrett Rd.
Dowagiac MI 49047
E-mail: lynjan@mich.com
Website: www.lynjan.com

(616) 424-6520
(616) 424-3475, fax

- Augmentative and alternative communication
- Curriculum adaptation
- Reading comprehension programs

Lynx
E-mail: lynxdev@browser.org
Website: http://lynx.browser.org

- Standard web browser

Maddak, Inc.
661 Route 23 S.
Wayne NJ 07470
E-mail: custservice@maddak.com
Website: www.maddak.com

(973) 628-7600
(973) 305-0841, fax

- Pointing and typing aids

*Madentec, Limited
4664 99 St.
Edmonton AB T6E 5H5
Canada
E-mail: techsup@madenta.com
Website: www.madentec.com

(877) 623-3682
(780) 450-8926
(780) 988-6182, fax

- Alternate keyboards
- On-screen keyboards
- Electronic aids to daily living
- Switch software
- Word prediction programs
- Electronic head-pointing device

*MarbleSoft
12301 Central Ave. NE
Blaine MN 55434
E-mail: mail@marblesoft.com
Website: www.marblesoft.com

(763) 755-1402
(763) 862-2920, fax

- Early-childhood software
- Reading comprehension programs
- Switch software

The Matias Corporation
129 Rowntree Dairy Rd., Unit #20

(888) 663-4263

Vaughan ON L4L 6E1
Canada
E-mail: info@half-qwerty.com
Website: http://half-qwerty.com
- Access utilities

(905) 265-8844

*Mayer-Johnson Company
PO Box 1579
Solana Beach CA 92075
E-mail: mayerj@mayer-johnson.com
Website: www.mayerjohnson.com
- Alternate keyboards
- Augmentative and alternative communication products
- Speech synthesizers
- Writing-composition programs
- Talking word processors

(800) 588-4548
(858) 550-0084
(858) 550-0449, fax

Maxess Products, Ltd.
The Chinestone, Dancers Hill
Charlbury, Oxfordshire OX7 3RZ
UK
E-mail: sales@maxessproducts.co.uk
Website: www.ukonline.co.uk/special access
- Keyguards

+44-1608-811909, phone, fax

MaxiAids
42 Executive Blvd.
Farmingdale NY 11735
E-mail: inquiries@maxiaids.com
Website: www.maxiaids.com
- CCTVs
- Visual aids
- Reading tools
- Products for the deaf and hard of hearing
- PDAs

(800) 522-6294
(631) 752-0521
(631) 752-0738, TTY
(631) 752-0689, fax

McGraw-Hill Children's Publishing
3195 Wilson Dr. NW
Grand Rapids MI 49544
Website: www.mhkids.com
- Reading comprehension programs

(800) 417-3261

Med Labs, Inc.
28 Vereda Cordillera
Goleta CA 93117

(800) 968-2486
(805) 968-2486, voice, fax

356

Computer
Resources
for People
with
Disabilities

E-mail: medlabsinc@aol.com
Website: http://hometown.aol.com/medlabsinc
- Switches
- Electronic aids to daily living

*Microsoft Accessibility
Microsoft Corporation   (800) 426-9400
1 Microsoft Way   (800) 892-5234, TTY
Redmond WA 98052
Website: www.microsoft.com/enable
- Access utilities
- Menu-management programs
- Trackballs
- Voice recognition
- Screen magnification programs

*MicroTalk
203 Pleasantview Ave.   (502) 721-9907
Louisville KY 40206   (502) 721-9709 fax
E-mail: support@microtalk.com
Website: www.microtalk.com
- Braille translators
- Screen readers
- Speech synthesizers

*Millenium Software
3155 Fujita St.   (310) 530-0356
Torrance CA 90505
E-mail: peuapeu@aol.com
Website: http://members.aol.com/peuapeu
- Cognitive-training software
- Reading comprehension programs

Milliken Publishing Company
11643 Lilburn Park Rd.   (800) 325-4136
St. Louis MO 63146   (314) 991-4220
E-mail: webmaster@millikenpub.com   (314) 991-4807, fax
Website: www.millikenpub.com
- Educational software
- Reading comprehension programs

Mindplay
440 S. Williams Blvd., Suite 206   (520) 888-1800
Tucson AZ 85711   (520) 888-7904, fax
E-mail: mail@mindplay.com

Website: www.mindplay.com
- Educational software
- Reading comprehension programs
- Writing-composition programs

Mobius Corporation
405 N. Henry St.
Alexandria VA 22314
E-mail: Kidware@prodigy.net
Website: www.kidware.com/mobius

(800) 426-2710
(703) 684-2919, fax

- Early-childhood software

NanoPac, Inc.
4823 South Sheridan Rd., Suite 302
Tulsa OK 74145-5717
E-mail: info@nanopac.com
Website: www.nanopac.com

(800) 580-6086
(918) 665-0329
(918) 665-2310, TTY
(918) 665-0361, fax

- Switch software
- Voice recognition
- Braille products
- Augmentative communication software
- Alternate keyboards
- Electronic aids to daily living

Neovision
E-mail: neovision@neovision.cz
Website: www.neovision.cz

- Optical Braille recognition

Netscape Communications Corporation
PO Box 7050
Mountain View CA 94039-7050
Website: channels.netscape.com

(650) 254-1900
(650) 528-4124, fax

- Standard web browsers

Nextel
2001 Edmund Halley Dr.
Reston VA 20191
Website: nextelonline.nextel.com

(800) 639-6111
(800) 639-8359

- Cell phones

Nisus Software, Inc.
PO Box 1300
Solana Beach CA 92075

(800) 890-3030
(858) 481-1477

358

Computer
Resources
for People
with
Disabilities

E-mail: info@nisus.com
Website: www.nisus.com
    • Access utilities

(858) 481-6154, fax

North Coast Medical, Inc.
18305 Sutter Blvd.
Morgan Hill CA 95037
E-mail: custserv@ncmedical.com
Website: www.ncmedical.com
    • Pointing and typing aids

(800) 821-9319
(408) 776-5000
(877) 213-9300, fax

NXI Communications
4505 South Wasatch Blvd., Suite 120
Eagle Plaza Center
Salt Lake City UT 84124
E-mail: nxi@nextalk.com
Website: www.nxicom.com
    • TTY modems

(801) 274-6001
(801) 274-6002, fax
(801) 274-6004, TTY

*OMS Development
1013 West 32nd St., Suite 1F
Chicago IL 60608
E-mail: ebohlman@omsdev.com
Website: www.omsdev.com
    • Screen readers
    • Word prediction programs

(773) 247-1632
(773) 247-1742, fax

Opera Software
2700 Pecan St. W., Suite 400
Pflugerville TX 78660
Website: www.opera.com
    • Standard browsers

(512) 990-4336

Optelec USA, Inc.
321 Billerica Rd.
Chelmsford MA 01824
E-mail: customerservice@optelec.com
Website: www.optelec.com
    • CCTVs
    • Screen magnification programs

(800) 828-1056
(800) 929-2444, fax

*Optimum Resource, Inc.
18 Hunter Rd.
Hilton Head Island SC 29926
E-mail: stickyb@stickybear.com

(888) 784-2592
(843) 689-8000
(843) 689-8008, fax

Website: www.stickybear.com
- Educational software
- Reading comprehension programs

ORCCA Technology
444 East Main St., Suite 101   (859) 226-9625
Lexington KY 40507   (859) 226-0936, fax
E-mail: orcca@orcca.com
Website: www.orcca.com
- Switches

Origin Instruments Corporation
854 Greenview Dr.   (972) 606-8740
Grand Prairie TX 75050-2438   (972) 606-8741, fax
E-mail: support@orin.com
Website: www.orin.com
- Electronic pointing devices

OVAC Magnification Systems
67-555 East Palm Canyon Dr.   (800) 325-4488
Building C-103   (760) 321-9220
Cathedral City CA 92234   (760) 321-9711, fax
E-mail: info@ovac.com
Website: www.ovac.com
- CCTVs

*PageMinder
10580 Barkley St., Suite 450   (888) 882-7787
Overland Park KS 66212   (913) 383-9800
E-mail: pageminder@pageminderinc.com   (913) 649-0384, fax
Website: www.pageminderinc.com
- Mobility products
- Paging systems

Papenmeier
F.H. Papenmeier GmbH & Co. KG   +49-2304-205-0
PO Box 1620, D-58211   +49-2304-205-205, fax
Schwerte, Germany
E-mail: info@papenmeier.de
Website: www.papenmeier.de
- Refreshable Braille display

Parrot
189 West 89th St., #12   (917) 441-7408
New York NY 10024

360

Computer
Resources
for People
with
Disabilities

E-mail: jj.grimaud@bluehandsfree.com
Website: www.parrot.fr
- Voice-activated PDA

Parrot Software
PO Box 250755
West Bloomfield MI 48325
E-mail: support@parrotsoftware.com
Website: www.parrotsoftware.com
- Cognitive-training software

(800) 727-7681
(248) 788-3223
(248) 788-3224, fax

*Pathways Development Group, Inc.
17409 57th Ave. W.
Lynnwood WA 98037
E-mail: mikea@pathwaysdg.com
Website: www.pathwaysdg.com
- Adaptive controls
- Game controls

(877) 742-4604
(425) 742-4674
(425) 745-9279, fax

Penny & Giles Computer Products, Ltd.
163 Pleasant St., Suite 4
Attleboro MA 02703
- Trackballs
- Joysticks

(508) 226-3008
(508) 226-5208, fax

Personal Data Systems, Inc.
PO Box 1008
Campbell CA 95009-1008
E-mail: info@personaldatasystems.com
Website: www.personaldatasystems.com
- Speech synthesizers

(408) 866-1126
(408) 866-1128, fax

Phone TTY, Inc.
1246 Route 46 W.
Parsippany NJ 07054-2121
E-mail: phonetty@aol.com
Website: www.phone-tty.com
- TTYs and TTY modems

(973) 299-6627
(973) 299-6626, TTY
(973) 299-7768, fax

Phonic Ear, Inc.
3880 Cypress Dr.
Petaluma CA 94954
E-mail: customerservice@phonicear.com
Website: www.phonicear.com
- Augmentative and alternative communication products

(800) 227-0735
(707) 769-1110
(707) 769-9624, fax

Potomac Technology

One Church St., Suite 101   (800) 433-2838, voice, TTY
Rockville MD 20850-4158   (301) 762-1892, fax
E-mail: info@potomactech.com
Website: www.potomactech.com
- TTYs
- Assistive listening devices

Premier Assistive Technology

13102 Blaisdell Dr.   (517) 668-8188
Dewitt MI 48820   (517) 668-2417, fax
E-mail: info@readingmadeeasy.com
Website: www.readingmadeeasy.com
- Reading machines

*Prentke Romich Company

1022 Heyl Rd.   (800) 262-1984
Wooster OH 44691   (330) 262-1984
E-mail: info@prentrom.com   (330) 263-4829, fax
Website: www.prentrom.com
- Alternate keyboards
- Augmentative and alternative communication products
- Electronic aids to daily living
- Electronic pointing devices
- Joysticks
- Keyboard additions
- Switches
- Word prediction programs

*Promedia

57 Lakeview Ave.   (800) 462-0930
Clifton NJ 07011   (973) 253-5601, fax
E-mail: promedia@mtlakes.csnet.net
Website: www.promedia-semerc.com
- Trackballs
- Joysticks
- Touch screens

Psychological Corporation

19500 Bulverde Rd.   (800) 872-1726
San Antonio TX 78259   (210) 339-5000
E-mail: customer_care@harcourt.com   (800) 232-1223, fax
Website: www.psychcorp.com
- Writing-composition programs

362

Computer
Resources
for People
with
Disabilities

Pulse Data HumanWare
175 Mason Circle   (800) 722-3393
Concord CA 94520   (925) 681-4630, fax
Website: www.humanware.com
- Braille embossers and translators
- CCTVs
- Note takers
- Refreshable Braille displays
- Screen magnification programs
- Screen readers
- Speech synthesizers
- PDAs

Quartet Technology, Inc.
87 Progress Ave.   (978) 649-4328
Tyngsboro MA 01879   (978) 649-8363, fax
E-mail: info@qtiusa.com
Website: www.qtiusa.com
- Electronic aids to daily living

Qwerks.com, Inc.
1648 Willow Dr.   (888) 282-5887
Kaysville UT 84037   (801) 444-2837
E-mail: support@qwerks.com   (801) 497-9456, fax
Website: www.qwerks.com
- Accessible browsers and add-ons

*Raised Dot Computing, Inc.
(see Duxbury Systems, Inc.)

RC Systems, Inc.
1609 England Ave.   (425) 355-3800
Everett WA 98203   (425) 355-1098, fax
E-mail: info@rcsys.com
Website: www.rcsys.com
- Speech synthesizers

*RehabTool.com
PO Box 572190   (281) 531-6106
Houston TX 77257
E-mail: info@rehabtool.com
Website: www.rehabtool.com
- Augmentative and alternative communication products
- Alternative access
- Bilingual voice output
- Voice recognition

Research in Motion
295 Phillip St.   (519) 888-7465
Waterloo ON N2L 3W8   (519) 888-7884, fax
Canada
E-mail: webinfo@rim.net
Website: www.rim.net
- Pagers

*Rhamdec, Inc.
Mydesc Division   (800) 469-3372
PO Box 4296   (408) 496-5590
Santa Clara CA 95056   (408) 496-5593, fax
E-mail: sales@mydesc.com
Website: www.rhamdec.com
- Computer mounting products

*Richard Wanderman
(see LD Resources)

*Riverdeep, Inc
500 Redwood Blvd.   (415) 763-4700
Novato CA 94947
E-mail: info@riverdeep.net
Website: www.riverdeep.net
- Educational software
- Menu-management programs
- Reading comprehension programs
- Switch software
- Touch screens
- Writing-composition programs
- Access utilities
- Augmentative and alternative communication products
- Electronic aids to daily living
- Screen magnification programs
- Word prediction programs

*R. J. Cooper and Associates
27601 Forbes Rd., Suite 39   (800) 752-6673
Laguna Niguel CA 92677   (949) 582-2749
E-mail: info@rjcooper.com   (949) 582-3169, fax
Website: www.rjcooper.com
- Alternate keyboards
- Interface devices
- Joysticks
- Switches and switch software

364

Computer
Resources
for People
with
Disabilities

Robotron Group
15 Stamford Rd.   +61-3-9568-2568
Oakleigh, Victoria 3166   +61-3-9568-1377, fax
Australia
Website: www.robogroup.com
  • Reading machines

*Roger Wagner Publishing, Inc.
(see Sunburst Technology Corporation)

*Saltillo Corporation
2143 TR 112   (330) 674-6722
Millersburg OH 44654   (330) 674-6726, fax
E-mail: aac@saltillo.com
Website: www.saltillo.com
  • Augmentative and alternative communication products
  • PDAs

Sammons Preston, Rolyan
An AbilityOne Company   (800) 323-5547
4 Sammons Ct.   (800) 325-1745, TTY
Bolingbrook IL 60440   (800) 547-4333, fax
E-mail: spr@abilityone.com
Website: www.sammonsprestonrolyan.com
  • Pointing and typing aids
  • Switches
  • Aids for daily living

Saunders Ergo Source
4250 Norex Dr.   (800) 456-1289
Chaska MN 55318   (800) 375-1119, fax
  • Arm and wrist supports

Scan Soft
9 Centennial Dr.   (800) 443-7077
Peabody MA 01960   (987) 977-2000
Website: www.scansoft.com
  • Optical character recognition software
  • Voice recognition

Schamex Research
19201 Parthenia St., Suite H   (818) 772-6644
Northridge CA 91324   (818) 993-2496, fax
  • Reading machines

Scholastic Software

2931 East McCarty St.   (800) 541-5513
Jefferson City MO 65102   (573) 636-5271
Website: www.scholastic.com
- Reading comprehension programs
- Writing-composition programs

Semerc/ProMedia

57 Lakeview Ave.   (800) 462-0930
Clifton NJ 07011   (973) 253-7600
E-mail: promedia@mtlakes.csnet.net   (973) 253-5601, fax
Website: www.promedia-semerc.com
- Educational software
- Switch software

*Sensory Software International

26 Abbey Rd.   +01684-578868
Malvern WR14 3HD   +01684-897753, fax
United Kingdom
E-mail: info@sensorysoftware.com
Website: www.sensorysoftware.com
- Switch software
- Augmentative and alternative communication products
- Writing-composition programs
- Talking word processor

Serotek Corporation

1128 Harmon Pl., Suite 310   (866) 202-0520
Minneapolis MN 55403   (612) 659-0760, fax
E-mail: support@freedombox.info
Website: www.freedombox.info
- Accessible browsers and add-ons

*Seventh Generation Technologies (7GT)

5902-F Gunbarrel Ave.   (800) 500-2921
Boulder CO 80301   (720) 841-6900
E-mail: Info@7GT.com
Website: www.7GT.com
- Speech/language-instruction software

Siboney Learning Group

325 N. Kirkwood Rd., Suite 200   (800) 351-1404
St. Louis MO 63122   (888) 726-8100
E-mail: support@siboneylg.com   (314) 984-8063, fax
Website: www.gamco.com
- Reading comprehension software

366

Computer
Resources
for People
with
Disabilities

Sighted Electronics, Inc.
69 Woodland Ave.   (800) 666-4883
Westwood NJ 07675
Website: www.sighted.com
  • CCTVs

Silent Call Communications
4581 S. Lapeer Rd., Suite F   (800) 572-5227, voice, TTY
Lake Orion MI 48359   (248) 377-4700, voice, TTY
E-mail: silentcall@silentcall.com   (248) 377-4168, fax
Website: www.silent-call.com
  • Products for the deaf and hard of hearing

Silicon Graphics, Inc. (SGI)
1600 Amphitheatre Pkwy.   (800) 800-SGI1 (800-7441)
Mountain View CA 94043   (650) 960-1980
Website: www.sgi.com
  • Access utilities

*Simtech Publications
22 Spring Hill Rd.   (866) 485-1052
Harwinton CT 06791-1701   (860) 485-1052
E-mail: switchdon@hsj.com
Website: www.hsj.com
  • Educational software
  • Switch software

Skills Bank Corporation
(see Riverdeep, Inc.)

SkiSoft Publishing Corporation
PO Box 634   (781) 863-1876
Lexington MA 02420
E-mail: info@skisoft.com
Website: www.skisoft.com
  • Large-print word processors

Slater Software
351 Badger Ln.   (877) 306-6968
Guffey CO 80820   (719) 479-2255
Website: www.slatersoftware.com   (719) 479-2254, fax
  • Writing-composition programs

SoftTouch
4300 Stine Rd., Suite 401   (877) 763-8868
Bakersfield CA 93313   (661) 396-8676

Website: www.softtouch.com
- Augmentative and alternative communication products
- Switch software

Sonic Alert, Inc
1050 East Maple Rd.	(248) 577-5400, voice, TTY
Troy MI 48083	(248) 577-5433, fax

E-mail: sonic-info@sonicalert.com
- Products for the deaf and hard of hearing

Span-America Medical Systems, Inc.
PO Box 5231	(800) 888-6752
Greenville SC 29606	(864) 288-8877
Website: http://spanamerica.com	(864) 288-8692, fax

- Keyboard additions
- Seating and positioning

*Special Needs Project Worldwide
3463 State St., Suite 282	(800) 333-6867
Santa Barbara CA 93105	(805) 962-8087
E-mail: books@specialneeds.com	(805) 962-5087, fax

Website: www.specialneeds.com
- Books

Speech and Braille Unlimited
E-mail: info@speechbraille.com	(612) 644-2052

Website: www.speechbraille.com
- Products for people who are blind or have low vision

*Spinoza Company
2666 Patton Rd.	(800) 282-2327
Roseville MN 55113-1136	(651) 604-6681, fax

E-mail: spinoza@spinozabear.com
Website: www.spinozabear.com
- Adapted toys

Sprint
6200 Sprint Pkwy.	(800) 829-0965
Overland Park KS 66251	

Website: www.sprint.com
- Cell phones
- Video-relay service

*SSB Technologies
1000 Sansome St., Suite 280	(415) 975-8000
San Francisco CA 94111	(415) 732-7508, fax

368

Computer
Resources
for People
with
Disabilities

E-mail: contact@ssbtechnologies.com
Website: www.ssbtechnologies.com
- Web accessibility testing tool

SSK Technology, Inc.
5619 Scotts Valley Dr., Suite 280
Scotts Valley CA 95066
E-mail: writalk@aol.com
- TTYs

(800) 775-0759
(800) 775-1630, TTY
(408) 461-8909, fax

*Sunburst Technology Corporation
1550 Executive Dr.
Elgin IL 60123
E-mail: service@sunburst.com
Website: www.sunburst.com
- Alternate keyboards
- Authoring software
- Educational software
- Large-print word processors
- Math software
- Reading comprehension programs
- Writing-composition programs

(800) 321-7511
(888) 800-3028

*Sun Microsystems Accessibility Program
2515 North First St.
San Jose CA 95131
E-mail: access@sun.com
Website: www.sun.com/access
- Internet accessibility
- Internet developer products

(408) 863-3151
(408) 863-3228

SVE and Churchill Media
6677 N. Northwest Hwy.
Chicago IL 60631
E-mail: CustServ@SVEmedia.com
Website: www.svemedia.com
- Reading comprehension programs
- Electronic reference tools

(800) 829-1900
(800) 624-1678
(773) 775-9550
(773) 775-5091, fax

Switch In Time
172 Harvard Rd.
Littleton MA 01460
E-mail: adams@switchintime.com
Website: www.switchintime.com
- Switches and switch software

(978) 486-9433

Sym Systems/The Great Talking Box Company
(see The Great Talking Box Company)

*TASH International, Inc.

3512 Mayland Ct.   (804) 747-5020
Richmond VA 23233   (804) 747-5224, fax
E-mail: tashinc@aol.com
Website: www.tashint.com

- Abbreviation expansion and macro programs
- Alternate keyboards
- Augmentative and alternative communication products
- Electronic aids to daily living
- Interface devices
- Joysticks
- Keyboard additions
- Switches and switch software

Taylor Associates Communications, Inc.

200-2 E. 2nd St.   (800) READ-PLUS (732-3758)
Huntington Station NY 11746   (631) 549-3000
E-mail: ifno@ta-comm.com   (631) 549-3156, fax
Website: www.ta-comm.com

- Reading comprehension-improvement programs
- Visual/functioning training

Teacher Support Software

3542 N. St.   (800) 228-2871
Gainesville FL 32605   (904) 332-6404
                                                (904) 332-6779, fax

- Reading comprehension programs
- Talking and large-print word processors
- Writing-composition programs

Tech-Able/Member Toy Adaptation Network for Children with Disabilities

1114 Brett Dr.   (770) 922-6768
Conyers GA 30094   (770) 922-6769, fax
E-mail: techweb@techable.org
Website: www.techable.org

- Keyguards
- Switches

Technology for Language and Learning

PO Box 327   (516) 625-4550

370

Computer
Resources
for People
with
Disabilities

East Rockaway NY 11518-0327 (516) 621-3321, fax
  • Switches and switch software

Technos America, Ltd. LLC
386 Quartz Circle (877) 816-0495
Bailey CO 80421 (303) 816-9006
E-mail: info@mctos.com (303) 816-9619, fax
Website: www.mctos.com
  • Electronic pointing devices
  • Switches, communication software

Tek-Talk
8224 E. Brandscreek Way (208) 724-6321
Nampa ID 83687 (208) 371-4213
E-mail: mwilson@tek-talk.net (208) 442-8966, fax
Website: www.tek-talk.net
  • Cell phones

Teledyne Brown Engineering/Interact Plus Division
2225 Drake Ave., Suite 2 (800) 944-8002
Huntsville AL 35805 (256) 880-8785, fax
E-mail: info@interactplus.com
Website: www.interactplus.com
  • Electronic aids to daily living

*Telesensory
520 Almanor Ave. (800) 804-8004
Sunnyvale CA 94085 (408) 616-8700
E-mail: info@telesensory.com (408) 616-8720, fax
Website: www.telesensory.com
  • Braille embossers, translators
  • CCTVs
  • Note takers
  • Reading machines
  • Refreshable Braille displays
  • Screen magnification programs
  • Screen readers
  • Speech synthesizers
  • TTYs
  • Browser access

Texas School for the Deaf
1102 South Congress Ave. (800) DEAF-TSD (332-4873), voice, TTY
PO Box 3538 (512) 462-5353, voice, TTY
Austin TX 78764

E-mail: ercod@tsd.state.tx.us
Website: www.tsd.state.tx.us/
- Educational software

*Texthelp Systems Ltd. (formerly Lorien Systems)

Enkalon Business Centre	(888) 333-9907 (U.S.)
25 Randalstown Rd.	(877) 631-6991, fax (U.S.)
Antrim BT41 4LJ	+44-28-9442-8105 (U.K. phone)
N. Ireland	

E-mail: info@texthelp.com
Website: www.texthelp.com
- Reading and writing software
- Accessible browsers and add-ons
- Word prediction programs
- Talking word processors

Thales Navigation

960 Overland Ct.	(800) 669-4477
San Dimas CA 91773	(909) 394-7070, fax

Website: www.magellangps.com
- Global positioning systems (GPS)

T-Mobile

PO Box 37380	(800) 937-8997
Albuquerque NM 87176-7380	

Website: www.t-mobile.com
- Cell phones

Tom Snyder Productions

80 Coolidge Hill Rd.	(800) 342-0236
Watertown MA 02172-2817	(800) 304-1254, fax

E-mail: ask@tomsnyder.com
Website: www.tomsnyder.com
- Educational software
- Reading comprehension programs
- Writing-composition programs

Toys for Special Children, Inc. (a subsidiary of Enabling Devices)

385 Warburton Ave.	(800) 832-8697
Hastings on Hudson NY 10706	(914) 478-0960
Website: www.enablingdevices.com	(914) 478-7030, fax

- Adapted toys
- Electronic aids to daily living
- Switches and switch software

372

Computer
Resources
for People
with
Disabilities

Trace Research and Development Center
University of Wisconsin at Madison   (608) 262-6966
2107 Engineering Centers Bldg.   (608) 263-5408, TTY
1550 Engineering Dr.   (608) 262-8848, fax
Madison WI 53706
E-mail: info@trace.wisc.edu
Website: http://trace.wisc.edu
- Information resources

Troll Touch
25530 Avenue Stanford, Suite 201   (661) 257-1160
Valencia CA 91355-1131   (661) 257-1161, fax
E-mail: info@trolltouch.com
Website: www.trolltouch.com
- Touch screens

Turning Point Therapy & Technology, Inc.
PO Box 310751   (877) 608-9812
New Braunfels TX 78131-0751   (830) 608-9812
E-mail: sales@turningpointtechnology.com   (830) 606-3810, fax
Website: www.turningpointtechnology.com
- Keyguards

*UCLA Intervention Program
1000 Veteran Ave., Rm. 23-10   (310) 825-4821
Los Angeles CA 90095-1797   (310) 206-7744, fax
Website: www.bol.ucla.edu/~kloo/IP/Home.htm
- Alternate-keyboard software
- Early-childhood software
- Intellikeys software
- Switches and switch software

Ultratec
450 Science Dr.   (800) 482-2424, voice, TTY
Madison WI 53711   (608) 238-5400, voice, TTY
Website: www.ultratec.com   (608) 238-3008, fax
E-mail: service@ultratec.com
- Payphone attachments
- Signaling equipment
- TTYs
- Products for the deaf and hard of hearing

UMAX Technologies, Inc.
10460 Brockwood Rd.   (214) 342-9799

Dallas TX 75238   (214) 342-9046, fax
E-mail: support@umaxcare.com
Website: www.umax.com
- Scanners

Varatouch Technology, Inc. (formerly Presentation Electronics)

7325 Roseville Rd.   (800) 888-9281
Sacramento CA 95842   (916) 331-6300
E-mail: mrogers@varatouch.com *or*   (916) 338-8255, fax
  jvillegas@varatouch.com
Website: www.varatouch.com
- Remote controls

Verizon

Website: www.verizon.com
- Cell phones

VideoEye! Corporation

10211 West Emerald   (800) 416-0758
Boise ID 83704   (208) 323-9577
Website: www.videoeyecorp.com   (208) 377-1528, fax
- CCTVs

Visioneer

5673 Gibraltar Dr., Suite 150   (925) 251-6398
Pleasanton CA 94588   (925) 416-8615, fax
Website: www.visioneer.com
- Scanners

Vision Technology Inc.

8501 Delport Dr.   (800) 560-7226
St. Louis MO 63114-5905   (314) 890-8300
E-mail: vti@vti1.com
Website: www.visiontechinc.com
- CCTVs

Visuaide, Inc.

841 Jean-Paul Vincent Blvd.   (888) 723-7273
Longueuil Quebec J4G1R3   (450) 463-1717
Canada   (450) 463-0120, fax
E-mail: info@visuaide.com
Website: www.visuaide.com
- Switches and switch software

Visual Tech Connection

PO Box 1996   (800) 589-8835

374

Computer
Resources
for People
with
Disabilities

8174 Rookery Way
Westerville OH 43086
- Monitor additions: magnifiers

Walker Equipment
4289 Bonny Oaks Dr., Suite 106   (800) 552-3368
Chattanooga TN 37406   (423) 622-7793
E-mail: product@mywalker.com   (423) 622-7646, fax
Website: www.mywalker.com
- Products for the deaf and hard of hearing

WCI Technology
Weitbrecht Communications, Inc.   (800) 233-9130, voice, TTY
2716 Ocean Park Blvd., Suite 1007   (310) 450-9918, fax
Santa Monica CA 90405
Website: www.weitbrechtcom.com
E-mail: sales@weitbrecht.com
- TTYs

*WesTest Engineering Corporation
810 W. Shepard Ln.   (801) 451-9191
Farmington UT 84025   (801) 451-9393, fax
E-mail: webmail@westest.com
Website: www.westest.com
- Interface devices

*William K. Bradford Publishing
35 Forest Ridge Rd.   (800) 421-2009
Concord MA 01742   (978) 318-9500, fax
E-mail: wkb@wkbradford.com
Website: www.wkbradford.com
- Reading comprehension programs
- Writing-composition programs

*Wizcom Technologies, Inc
257 Great Rd.   (888) 777-0552
Acton MA 01720   (978) 929-9228, fax
E-mail: info@wizcomtech.com
Website: www.wizcomtech.com
- Handheld scanner
- Electronic reference tool

Words+, Inc.
1220 West Ave. J   (800) 869-8521
Lancaster CA 93534-2902   (661) 723-6523

E-mail: info@words-plus.com
Website: www.words-plus.com

(661) 723-2114, fax

- Access utilities
- Alternate keyboards
- Augmentative and alternative communication products
- Electronic pointing devices
- Electronic aids to daily living
- Interface devices
- Keyguards
- Switches and switch software
- Word prediction programs
- Abbreviation expansion and macros

Wynd Communications Corporation
75 Higuera St., Suite 240
San Luis Obispo CA 93401
E-mail: info@wynd.com
Website: www.wynd.com

(800) 549-9800
(800) 549-2800, TTY
(805) 781-6001, fax

- Accessible pagers

Xerox Imaging Systems, Inc.
9 Centennial Dr.
Peabody MA 01960
Website: www.xerox.com

(800) 275-9376
(508) 977-2000
(508) 977-2148

- Optical character recognition software
- Reading machines

XYBIX Systems, Inc.
8160 Blakeland Dr., Unit G
Littleton CO 80125
E-mail: info@xybix.com
Website: www.xybix.com

(800) 788-2810
(303) 683-5656
(303) 683-5454, fax

- Arm and wrist supports
- Adaptable furniture

YoMax Communications
5711 E. Waltann Ln.
Scottsdale AZ 85254
E-mail: support@yomax.com
Website: www.yomax.com

(800) 808-0966
(602) 996-7434
(602) 493-0262, fax

- Pagers

Zygo Industries, Inc.
PO Box 1008
Portland OR 97207-1008

(800) 234-6006
(503) 684-6006

376

———

Computer
Resources
for People
with
Disabilities

E-mail: zygo@zygo-usa.com

(503) 684-6011, fax

Website: www.zygo-usa.com

- Alternate keyboards
- Augmentative and alternative communication products
- Electronic aids to daily living
- Switches and switch software

Keyword Index

Because disabilities vary in both impact and degree, we have found that it is sometimes useful to research information by specific limitation. For example, someone with multiple sclerosis may have obvious issues related to dexterity—such as the physical ability to use a keyboard or mouse—but may also have subtler or longer-term needs related to their vision or speech. The Keyword Index is provided so you can look up information based on categories of functional limitation. It is intended to assist readers in accessing the information contained in this book in ways that are relevant to their specific goals and most immediate questions.

The Keyword Index may also be useful if you are dealing with a temporary functional limitation or a situation related to an environmental limitation. For example, some of the technologies listed under the keyword "Physical" may be useful for someone with a broken finger or wrist, and some of the technologies listed under "Blindness" may be useful for photographers, spelunkers, and others who work in dark environments.

Once you have determined your relevant needs and turned to the appropriate keyword, you will find four subcategories of information:

Stories/Life Situations. This subcategory points you to specific examples of how people with the functional limitation you're searching under have chosen and used assistive technology; it also points you to information about special considerations that may be relevant based upon an individual's specific life circumstances.

Example: Under the keyword "Blindness," the Stories/Life Situations index refers you to stories about how people who lack any ability to read from a monitor have explored alternative output methods. It also refers you to appropriate sections of the book that address various life situations (e.g., various ages or goals).

Products. This subcategory lists relevant products and refers you to information about locating and contacting manufacturers of the products.

Example: Under the keyword "Learning," the Products index refers you to information about products designed for or useful for people with learning disabilities.

Resources. Whereas Part III lists many websites, organizations, and other information sources about assistive technology, this subcategory points you to resources specifically focused on the type(s) of functional limitations you're interested in.

KEYWORD INDEX

378

Computer
Resources
for People
with
Disabilities

Example: Under the keyword "Cognitive," the Resources index refers you to organizations and publications specifically relevant to people with cognitive or social-functioning limitations.

Charts. This subcategory points you to the "Ask Yourself" Chart (pp. 169–175) that is most likely to be of use to you. Keep in mind that the "Ask Yourself" Charts primarily refer to computer access technologies. Because the book doesn't include charts relevant to all types of functional limitations, some keywords don't list a "Charts" subcategory.

Example: Under the keyword "Low Vision," the Charts index refers you to the "Ask Yourself" Charts appropriate for researching options related to visual limitations.

Sample Searches

The parents of *Juanita*, a child with cerebral palsy, note that in a classroom setting she is able to use a standard Macintosh computer keyboard effectively, if slowly, but has major difficulties using the standard mouse. It isn't clear whether this is entirely due to her moderate spasticity or if her mild cognitive disability may also be a factor. In preparation for Juanita's next IEP meeting, her parents decide to look at information listed in the Keyword Index under both "Physical" and "Cognitive." This leads them to the "Ask Yourself" Charts that provide responses to the questions "How effectively can I use the mouse?" and "How effectively can I handle computer equipment?" For each of the two keywords, they then look under the subcategory "Resources" to obtain contact information for organizations they can consult about solutions that have worked for other children.

Noam, an adult with partial quadriplegia, already knows something about assistive technology. Now he wants to research appropriate job accommodations for computer use, including speech-input technology, on-screen keyboards, and word prediction, in more detail. Under the keyword "Physical," he looks under both Products and Stories/Life Situations for relevant tips about using these products in the workplace.

Chih-Hao, a 77-year-old man recovering from a recent stroke, asks two family members for help in purchasing a new computer. While discussing his request, one family member notes that Chih-Hao now only seems to have use of his left hand, and the other family member comments that he also appears to have significant difficulty reading a newspaper. To get an idea of what might be available to meet Chih-Hao's access needs, they use the Keyword Index to look under "Low Vision" and "Physical" and then at the subcategories "Resources" and "Products."

Note: *Software* refers to programs used on computers or computer-like devices. *Hardware* may indicate either technology used to improve computer accessibility or stand-alone devices used to improve general access to the user's environment.

Blindness

Information for individuals who are unable to view a standard computer monitor. Because most of these individuals will also be unable to use a standard mouse, this category covers both monitor alternatives and mouse alternatives. (Information for individuals who have some ability to view the monitor is listed under "Low Vision.")

Stories/Life Situations

Paula, 104

Products

Access utilities, 187

Braille embossers and translators, 235

Browsers and browser add-ons, 218

Keyboard additions, 190

Note takers, 31, 261

Optical character recognition and scanners, 203

Personal digital assistants (PDAs), 272

Reading machines and scan/read programs, 29, 263

Refreshable Braille displays, 238

Screen readers, 243

Software features, 176–180

Speech synthesizers, 240

Wireless products (cell phones, pagers, GPS), 266

Resources

ADA technology resources, 293

Organizations, 297, 299, 300 (Lighthouse), 302

Publications, 310, 311

Websites, listserves, and discussion lists, 320

380

Computer
Resources
for People
with
Disabilities

Charts

Cognitive

Information for individuals who have below-average or impaired intelligence or social functioning. This category covers both technology that may make computer use easier and technology that may assist with daily living skills. (Information for individuals who have average or above-average intelligence and social functioning but have difficulty with reading, writing, or mathematics is listed under "Learning.")

Stories/Life Situations

Products

Hearing

Information for individuals who have difficulty hearing or are unable to hear auditory feedback from the computer or from other technologies (e.g., telephones).

Stories/Life Situations

Products

382

Computer
Resources
for People
with
Disabilities

Learning

Information for individuals who have average or above-average intelligence and social functioning but have difficulty with the basic skills of reading, writing, or mathematics. This category covers technologies that provide assistance with computer use and with implementation of these skills in academic, work, or personal settings. (Information for individuals who have below-average or impaired intelligence or social functioning is listed under "Cognitive.")

Stories/Life Situation

Products

Low Vision

Information for individuals who have some ability to view a standard computer monitor. This category covers technology that makes on-screen information easier to view. (Information for individuals who are unable to view a standard computer monitor is listed under "Blindness.")

384

Computer
Resources
for People
with
Disabilities

Physical

Information for individuals who have difficulty moving, who have pain, or who are unable to use their hands, arms, shoulders, neck, or back when writing or accessing the computer mouse and/or keyboard. This category covers accessories (hardware and software) that can be used with the standard keyboard and mouse, as well as alternative keyboards and mice.

Stories/Life Situation

Products

Resources

Charts

Speech

Information for individuals who have physical and/or cognitive difficulties with communication. This category primarily covers augmentative and alternative communication (AAC) aids.

Stories/Life Situation

Anthony, 43

Chris, 9, 12

Early childhood, 17

James, 35

Leah, 15

Makenzie, 83

Melinda, 62

Pedro, 47

Tommy, 90

Products

Augmentative/alternative communication (AAC), 42, 43, 251

Switches and switch software, 83, 193

Talking photo albums, 87

Resources

Conferences and other events, 308

Funding requirements, 74

International resources, 307

Organizations, 296, 297, 299, 303

Publications, 310, 311, 313, 314

Index

A

GET FIT WHILE YOU SIT: Easy Workouts from Your Chair

by Charlene Torkelson

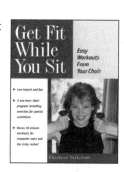

Here is a total-body workout that can be done right from your chair, anywhere. It is perfect for office workers and those with age-related movement limitations or special conditions. The One-Hour Chair Program is a full-body, low-impact workout that includes light aerobics and exercises to be done with or without weights. The 5-Day Short Program features five compact workouts for those short on time and the Ten-Minute Miracles are easy-to-do exercises perfect for doing at work.

160 pages ... 210 photos ... Paperback $14.95

COPING WITH VISION LOSS: Maximizing What You Can See and Do

by Bill Chapman, Ed.D., Foreword by Dr. Lin Moore

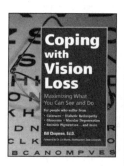

This book delivers on a special promise: People with severe vision loss can be helped and equipped to function as sighted. The author has a visual acuity of 20/240 but can read, use a computer without a voice synthesizer, and watch TV from 12 feet away, and he has driven 700,000 miles as a legally blind but licensed driver. He explains fundamental facts about eyes, vision, and vision rehab, including the varieties of diseases that destroy vision, skills that the partially sighted person must learn, and the best low vision aids available.

304 pages ... 29 illus. ... Paperback $16.95

I-CAN'T-CHEW COOKBOOK: Delicious Soft-Diet Recipes for People with Chewing, Swallowing and Dry-Mouth Disorders ... *by J. Randy Wilson*

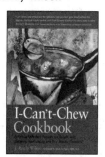

About 40 million people in the U.S. suffer from disorders that require them to eat soft foods, such as people who have TMJ problems; patients of stroke, cancer, ALS, Alzheimer's, AIDS, and lupus; and people recovering from serious surgery. The *I-Can't-Chew Cookbook* features 168 tasty and nutritious soft- or liquid-diet recipes with nutritional analysis and tips on preparation. Endorsed by a wide range of medical professionals, it contains a chapter by a registered dietician and is also available in a lie-flat spiral binding.

224 pages ... Paperback $16.95 ... Spiral bound $22.95

To order or receive a FREE catalog see next page or call (800) 266-5592

ORDER FORM

10%   DISCOUNT on orders of $50 or more —
20%   DISCOUNT on orders of $150 or more —
30%   DISCOUNT on orders of $500 or more —
On cost of books for fully prepaid orders

NAME

ADDRESS

CITY/STATE   ZIP/POSTCODE

PHONE   COUNTRY (outside of U.S.)

TITLE	QTY	PRICE	TOTAL
Computer Resources for People ... (paper)		@ $24.95	
Computer Resources for People ... (spiral)		@ $31.95	

Prices subject to change without notice

Please list other titles below:

		@ $	
		@ $	
		@ $	
		@ $	
		@ $	

Check here to receive our book catalog ☐   *FREE*

Shipping Costs:
By Priority Mail, first book $4.50, each additional book $1.00
By UPS and to Canada, first book $5.50, each additional book $1.50
For rush orders and other countries call us at (510) 865-5282

TOTAL _____
Less discount @ _____ %   (_____)
TOTAL COST OF BOOKS _____
Calif. residents add 7½ sales tax _____
add Shipping & handling _____
TOTAL ENCLOSED _____
Please pay in U.S. funds only

☐ Check   ☐ Money Order   ☐ Visa   ☐ MasterCard   ☐ Discover

Card # _____   Exp. date _____

Signature _____

Complete and mail to:
Hunter House Inc., Publishers
PO Box 2914, Alameda CA 94501-0914
Phone (510) 865-5282 Fax (510) 865-4295
You can also order by calling **(800) 266-5592**
of from **www.hunterhouse.com**

CTS4 ... 9/2004